PICKLES
&
ICE
CREAM

Here are some thoughts on
Pickles and Ice Cream
from readers like you...

...*Pickles and Ice Cream* is a comprehensive guide to pregnancy, informative, well-written and witty. The trimester format makes locating information easy. I found this book to be a great source of general pregnancy information for moms-to be too. Every expectant couple should have a copy! —*Karen Russo-Stieglitz, MD,*
Maternal-Fetal Medicine Specialist.

...the book provided me with insights into being a better husband during my wife's pregnancy. Dr. B's book is an easy read and packed full of interesting and helpful information. I highly recommend it to all fathers-to-be.
—*Dan O.*

...*Pickles and Ice Cream* provides the perfect balance of no-nonsense practical advice, humor and clarification of so many of the "mysteries" experienced during those precious nine months....

—*Neal P.*

...Even though I have numerous maternity texts, I turn to *Pickles and Ice Cream* for the right answer fast. I can't tell you how comforting it is to find reasonable, calming advice on so many issues about pregnancy. I know the book was written for soon-to-be fathers but this is one soon-to-be mom who feels much better informed because of your efforts. Thanks for your hard work....

—*Beth P.*

...It's a great book! *Pickles and Ice Cream* is far better than those lengthy maternity books and to the point. I liked the way Dr. Bissinger organized the book by trimester and alphabetical order....

—*Ken and Brenda C.*

...A must for my sons-in-laws during my daughters' pregnancies....

—*Lynne G.*

ACKNOWLEDGMENTS

Pickles and Ice Cream: A Father's Guide to Pregnancy could never have been written without the enthusiasm and quest for knowledge of my patients and their partners. Constantly questioning the mysteries of pregnancy, they provided me with all the material for this book. I am deeply indebted to them for trusting me with their care during this special time in their lives. Thanks go to them and to the many couples who reviewed the manuscript, helping to perfect each answer.

I am greatly appreciative of the efforts of Laura Kohler, Hillary Iggy-Post, and Carol Albright, who shared their editorial expertise and critical eye to help the project become a reality. The contributions of Drs. Christine Ganitsch, Scott Roseff, Ellen Williams, RN, and Beth DiGiacinto as readers and critics, helped ensure the project's success. Thanks also go to Kyle Godfrey, who's youthful but insightful words gave birth to the book's title.

My greatest appreciation and respect go to my art director, Robin Arzt, and editor, Marilyn Knowlton for the professionalism and fantastic effort. Without their guidance, *Pickles and Ice Cream* would never have found its way out of my waiting room.

I want to recognize and thank Dr. Todd Rosen, Director of Atlantic Health System's Department of Maternal-Fetal Medicine, who offered his erudite comments and incredible wealth of knowledge to ensure the accuracy of the information provided.

Professionally, I have been blessed with three terrific partners: David Hirsch, Dawn Goldstein, and Stephen Leviss. Together we have shared nearly twenty years of joy, caring for our patients and bringing happiness to thousands of our neighbors. Their support and insights have helped me become a better person and physician. To them, I say thank you for opening your hearts and lives to me and my family.

My second professional family—the nurses and staff at Morristown Memorial Hospital's Labor and Delivery and Mother-Baby Unit—are truly the unsung heroes! Without their tireless efforts and constant support, I would not be able to provide my patients with the best in obstetrical care. Thank you! I am grateful for the opportunity to work with such fine professionals on a daily basis.

My family has been my biggest support throughout the writing of this book. Their love and support have sustained and motivated me to make *Pickles and Ice Cream* the best book of its kind. Josh, Scott, and Lindsey, thanks for being my biggest fans. I love you very much!

As you can imagine, the spouse of an obstetrician must have a heart of gold. I am blessed with a truly extraordinary wife and partner, Margie. Her strength and conviction convinced me to create *Pickles and Ice Cream*. Her careful reading, gentle suggestions, and maternal insights gave the book its unique and powerful voice. I am a lucky man to have her. I love you, and thank you for helping create the book.

PICKLES
&
ICE
CREAM

*A Father's
Guide to
Pregnancy*

CRAIG BISSINGER, MD

To our Readers,
Our understanding of obstetrics is constantly changing.
This book is not intended to be an alternative to, or a substitute for, your own doctor's recommendations. It serves as a supplement to the information provided by your doctor.

Book design by Robin Arzt
Edited by Marilyn Knowlton

Library of Congress Control Number: 2003107278
Copyright © 2006 by Craig Bissinger, MD
Fourth printing

Workfit Consultants, L.L.C.
50 Cherry Hill Road, Suite 303
Parsippany, NJ 07054

Printed in Canada

CONTENTS

INTRODUCTION

Congratulations! There is a baby on the way. During the next nine months, you and your partner will need to prepare for one of life's most interesting adventures: parenthood. Your journey may not be quite as simple or straight-forward as you may think. There are decisions to make, tests to undergo, and a baby relying upon your judgments.

Life will change dramatically for your partner. Her mind and body are being rented by a welcome visitor, the grow-ing baby with its own unique set of demands. Her energy is being utilized to make kidneys, lungs, a heart, and all the other critical parts of your baby. While your partner's body works away, she needs to sleep more, her body's aching, and she is craving pickles and ice cream NOW!

As a practicing obstetrician, I have witnessed thousands of couples navigate the trials and tribulations of pregnancy. While many of my patients become avid readers, scouring every pregnancy book available to verify their symptoms, fathers-to-be most often prefer a concise guide. To help you be an understanding and helpful partner, I have written *Pickles and Ice Cream: A Father's Guide to Pregnancy*. This book provides to-the-point explanations of the many and varied symptoms and worries of pregnant couples, as well as a discussion of the standard tests and their implications.

For easy reference I have divided the book into four sections. Each section addresses a specific portion of the pregnancy and its most common concerns. As this is a brief guide, there will be some topics that are not discussed in this book. If you desire still more information on these issues, there are a variety of comprehensive pregnancy manuals available in your local bookstore and library, or you can speak with your partner's doctor.

Looking forward, there are many exciting moments to come: the first time you hear your baby's heart beat, seeing your baby on the ultrasound monitor, and feeling the baby kick are just a few examples. Each of these milestones will bring you and your partner closer to each other and to becoming a family. It won't always be smooth sailing, but together you will make your collective dream come true.

Sometimes you will feel quite alone on your journey, but you are not. Your friends and family are eager to reassure and comfort you. And we are with you too, quietly behind the scene, watching and admiring nature's handiwork at its finest. If you still have doubts, think about the caveman. He didn't have *Pickles and Ice Cream: A Father's Guide to Pregnancy*, and he managed! Relax and enjoy the next nine months.

Good luck,
Dr. B

FIRST TRIMESTER

The first three months are filled with strange new sensations. Your partner is noticing changes in her body and the way she feels. Sore breasts, bloating, nausea, and fatigue are just the tip of the iceberg. Her clothes are beginning to feel snug, and there are seven more months to go. She's craving the most bizarre foods and acting a bit odd. Be patient. She is making a baby, and it is hard work. Even she may be surprised by the many changes she is going through. Your developing baby is also going through a remarkable process as we speak. Its nervous system is sprouting and its heart is beating for the first time. Blood is beginning to circulate as the baby develops its lungs, kidneys, arms, and legs.

While you and your partner's dream of parenthood start to come into focus, there is an extended family already beaming with pride and excitement. Mom, Dad, Grandma, and Grandpa are reliving their sweet memories of youth and the awesome experience of becoming a parent. They know something special, and over the coming months you will begin to understand the great journey ahead.

HOW DO WE CONFIRM PREGNANCY?—Your partner should take a home pregnancy test when she is late. Although the various manufacturers promise 99 percent accuracy, the tests are less precise and may give a false negative result if done too soon. To ensure accuracy, wait five to seven days after a missed period.

> If the test is positive, save some money and don't buy another kit. She is pregnant. ***Congratulations!***

CALCULATING THE DUE DATE—You can make a good guess about the due date by using this simple formula. Take the date of the first day of the last menstrual period, subtract three months, and add seven days. This will give you the approximate due date. Typical pregnancies last from thirty-eight to forty-two weeks, or 269 days from ovulation.

> ***Example:***   Last period 4/14/00
> – 3 months
> +7 days
> **= Due date of 1/21/01**

> The precise due date may change if your partner's cycle deviates from the standard 28-day menstrual cycle.

HOW FAR ALONG IS MY PARTNER?—Most women remember the beginning of their last menstrual period better than the day they became pregnant. Because of this reality, obstetricians calculate how far along the pregnancy is by starting from the last menstrual period. By this method, the pregnancy will appear to last forty weeks, or ten months. So when I tell a patient she is eight weeks pregnant, I am telling her that the fetus is six weeks since conception and eight weeks since her last period. *Let's get this point straight up front.* Otherwise, it will drive both of you crazy for nine months. Also, every pregnancy book is geared to this method of calculating the length of pregnancy.

TERMS TO KNOW

If you want to be conversant in pregnancy lingo, here are the words to know in the first three months.

Abdominal ultrasound machine—A probe placed on the pregnant woman's stomach that uses sound waves to enable you to view the baby on a monitor. This test is performed to check for the baby's heartbeat and location. It is more accurate if performed after the seventh week of pregnancy.

Cervix—The opening of the uterus. It holds the baby inside. (Think of it as a door that remains shut until labor.)

Chorionic Villus Sampling (CVS)—A test performed at ten weeks of pregnancy to detect genetic abnormalities in the baby.

Due date or estimated date of confinement (EDC)—The predicted date of delivery.

Embryo—The growing baby in the first eight weeks of pregnancy.

Fetal heart tone—The baby's heartbeat.

Fetus—The growing baby after the first eight weeks of pregnancy.

Last menstrual period (LMP)—The first day of the last period. It is used to calculate the due date.

Midwife—A nurse trained to deliver babies vaginally.

Obstetrician—A licensed doctor trained to deliver babies vaginally and surgically.

Placenta—The fetal tissue attached to the uterus that exchanges food, oxygen, and fluid between the mother and baby.

Prenatal vitamins—Prescription-strength vitamins specifically composed and prescribed for pregnant women.

Transvaginal ultrasound machine—A probe placed in the vagina that uses sound waves to view the baby. This would be utilized before seven weeks of pregnancy or when an abdominal ultrasound fails to detect the baby or its heartbeat.

Trimester—One third of the pregnancy, each third being approximately thirteen weeks long.

Umbilical cord—Long tubular structure carrying blood vessels that connect the fetus to the placenta. Food, oxygen, and fluid are exchanged between the mother and baby through the cord.

Uterus—The organ holding the baby, also known as the womb.

While this is a brief list, it should enable you to keep up with your partner's new vocabulary.

Don't forget about me!

Throughout the pregnancy, there is a tendency for everyone to shower your partner with attention. This is a good thing. She needs all that positive reinforcement. Don't be surprised when your thoughts and feelings are ignored. After all, you are not carrying the baby. In fact, you have precious little to do with the pregnancy from this point on! This may be the truth, but you do have a lot on your plate. Your partner and your life are changing forever. It is for an amazing reason, but nonetheless, life will never be the same. There are philosophical questions to deal with. Will I make it through this ordeal? Can I deal with her special needs and still be my own man? Even more worrisome is the question, Will I be a good father? If you are asking yourself these questions, I can assure you the answer is "Yes" to all. You will be a great father.

Many fathers-in-waiting start to worry about the financial responsibility of parenthood. We tend to think more about college educations, but there is a considerable monetary commitment before that time. There are diapers, formula, a crib, clothes, and many other necessities to buy. Don't forget the baseball mitt, soccer cleats, ballet outfits, and stuffed animals. Say good-bye to your two-door sports car and get ready to embrace a station wagon or minivan. Don't get too worked up. My minivan can really scoot.

THE FIRST DOCTOR'S APPOINTMENT—This visit should be scheduled when your partner is between six and eight weeks from her last period. Attending this visit is a perfect time to support your partner. She will have an examination to confirm the pregnancy. In addition, time will be devoted to discussing the health history of both sides of the baby's family. Answers to these questions give the doctor insight into specific congenital conditions that might affect the pregnancy. Hemophilia, Tay-Sachs disease, cystic fibrosis, and sickle-cell anemia are some examples of medical conditions passed on from generation to generation. Before you even see the doctor, it is a good idea for you and your partner to become familiar with your families' health histories.

During this initial visit, the doctor will also discuss pregnancy issues such as dietary restrictions, activity, and exercise, as well as the upcoming standard blood testing (see *First lab tests* on page 14), office policies, and a schedule of office visits to monitor the pregnancy. Expect your partner to have monthly checkups until the twenty-eighth week, two- or three-week appointments until thirty-six weeks, and weekly visits thereafter. Make allowances in your schedule to attend some of the appointments. Your partner will appreciate your interest, and it gives you an opportunity to be involved. It can be very exciting to hear what is going on! In addition, an office visit is a great opportunity to get to know your partner's obstetrician.

Most men are not familiar with the obstetrician/gynecologist and the critical role he or she plays in making your collective birth experience safe and enjoyable. In many cases, your partner has an established relationship with the doctor. This brings a certain sense of comfort and security to this trusting relationship, which you have not had the opportunity to share. Now it is your turn to gain confidence in his or her skills as both a doctor and an educator.

Our role as doctor requires us to order and interpret test results, as well as to carefully monitor the pregnancy. Along the way we may suggest other tests to help determine the baby's health. We hope, as you get to know us, that you will develop the same level of trust that your partner has established with us. Our job doesn't end with test interpretation and the medical management of the pregnancy. We are an excellent educational resource for you and your partner. I would estimate that over half of each office visit is spent sharing information on what to expect when pregnant. This is the information that will help you and your partner answer those nagging questions that come up as the pregnancy progresses. This is precisely why I have written *Pickles and Ice Cream: A Father's Guide to Pregnancy*.

This forty-week adventure eventually comes to an end. When labor begins, you are embarking on a new course. You will put all your faith in this doctor/educator, hoping she or he will do a great job. Having developed trust and confidence in advance will help ease your concerns during this joyous yet stressful time.

So take my advice and meet the doctor(s).

FIRST LAB TESTS—Your partner will have some blood tests performed to screen for treatable medical conditions. These tests include a complete blood count; hepatitis B, syphilis, and rubella (German measles) testing; antibody screening; and a blood type. HIV testing and a urinalysis are included in the first lab tests. Abnormal results can lead to medical problems for your partner and baby. Fortunately, once identified, treatment can prevent a potential problem.

COMPLETE BLOOD COUNT—Testing to determine if your partner has a low blood count (anemia). With less blood available to carry oxygen, the baby's growth and development may be hindered. I suggest that my anemic patients use iron supplements with an added stool softener. Additional blood tests to screen for hereditary blood conditions such as sickle-cell anemia or thalasemia (Mediterranean anemia) will be ordered based upon the blood count and certain ethnic considerations. Nearly 8 percent of the African American population carries the trait for sickle-cell anemia (see *Genetic anemia* on page 18).

HEPATITIS B—A positive test indicates an infection in the mother's liver that can be transmitted to the baby during pregnancy or birth. Infected babies can develop a life-threatening liver infection. Vulnerable babies are treated with a shot of medicine at delivery to reduce their chances of developing hepatitis B. The American Academy of Pediatrics recommends that all babies receive a series of vaccines against hepatitis B beginning at birth and extending over the next six months. This is intended to prevent your baby from contracting this illness in the future.

SYPHILIS—A positive test suggests the presence of this sexually transmitted disease, which can cause medical problems for the mother and the newborn. Occasionally the first test is falsely positive. Therefore, we always order a confirming test to verify the results before initiating the strong antibiotic treatment needed by the mother. The medication is also effective for treating the baby. If your partner has syphilis, you should seek medical attention, since in all likelihood you also carry the infection and require treatment.

RUBELLA—This test determines your partner's risk for German measles. A woman with a negative test is considered susceptible. If she becomes infected with the virus, her baby may also become infected. Although rubella is a mild disease in adults, it causes severe birth defects in up to 50 percent of the infected babies! Susceptible women should be aware of their vulnerability and avoid children with an active infection or children who have not been vaccinated. Your partner should be vaccinated after delivery and can safely breast-feed. Vaccination should not be performed within three months of a planned pregnancy or during pregnancy. Although the consequences of this condition are bleak, this infection is incredibly rare in the United States because nearly every child is vaccinated against rubella.

BLOOD TYPE—The mother's blood type can be either A, B, AB, or O.

RH—The Rh test is done to determine whether the mother's blood type is positive or negative. If your partner is one of the 15 percent of women who are negative, she will receive a shot of Rhogam if she has an amniocentesis, at twenty-eight weeks of pregnancy, and after delivery, assuming the baby is Rh positive. Treatment is needed to prevent your partner from developing hostile antibodies to the baby's blood. Rh-positive women require no special treatment (see *Rh incompatability* on page 61).

ANTIBODY SCREEN—The test checks your partner's blood for potential allergies to the baby's blood cells. If this test is positive, the physician will suggest further evaluation.

HIV—A viral infection that will develop into AIDS. A positive test requires further evaluation to verify the accuracy of the test. Women carrying the virus should be put on medication during pregnancy to help prevent passage of the virus to their unborn child.

URINALYSIS—A sample of urine used to screen for kidney disease and infection. A urine culture is performed for those suspected of having an infection. A positive culture requires antibiotics to eradicate a urinary infection.

GENETIC SCREENING TESTS—Depending on your ethnic background, certain screening tests might be ordered.

> *Cystic fibrosis*—A serious medical condition that affects the baby's long-term health and life expectancy. Most physicians offer screening to all

couples of white northern European background, Ashkenazi Jewish people, those whose partner has cystic fibrosis, or those with a family history of the disease. Recent advances in technology have made testing a consideration for African American and Hispanic populations. The results are not quite as accurate as the test for the above-mentioned groups, but they still detect the majority of carriers. If the test is deemed appropriate, it will be ordered as part of your partner's initial lab tests. If she carries the gene, you will be checked by the same blood test. You both must have the gene in order to pass it on to your baby.

Jewish heritage diseases—A set of blood tests is used to screen for a series of serious genetic conditions including Tay-Sachs disease, Canavan, mucolipiddosis type IV, Gaucher's disease, Nieman-Pick, cystic fibrosis, Fanconi's Anemia, Bloom, and Familial Dysautonomia—all of which are prevalent among Ashkenazi Jewish people. Testing is recommended if both you and your partner are Jewish. First I ask the father to have his blood drawn to screen for these genetic conditions. The lab finds it easier to perform the screening on the man's blood rather than on his pregnant partner's protein-enriched blood, which can lead to inaccurate results. If you carry a gene for one of these conditions, your partner should also be tested. If you both have the same gene, 25 percent of your children will be affected with the disease. Genetic counseling and amniocentesis are recommended in this circumstance.

I am frequently asked if the testing should be done when only one partner is Jewish. My policy is to always screen the couple. I'd rather be safe in this instance.

Genetic anemia—Numerous blood conditions that can be passed on from couples of African, Indian, Arab, or Mediterranean descent to their baby. A screening test will be ordered on your partner as part of her initial lab testing. If she carries the gene, your blood will then be checked. These anemic conditions can only be passed on when you and your partner both carry the gene.

PRENATAL SCREENING—*First-trimester nuchal translucency and blood testing.*

Just when you have settled into the pregnancy routine, it is time to exercise some parental judgment. You have to make your first decision regarding testing to check if your baby has a serious problem such as Down syndrome. If your partner will be less than thirty-five years old when the baby is due, she is a candidate for a new screening test. Performed between the 11th and 14th week, this combination of several blood tests and an ultrasound measurement of the thickness of the skin over the baby's neck (nuchal translucency) is used to calculate the baby's risk of having Down syndrome. The test detects more than 80 percent of babies with this problem, as well as 20 percent of babies with heart abnormalities. If you have an abnormal test, your provider will suggest either a chorionic villus sampling (see *Chorionic Villus Sampling* on page 26) or an amniocentesis (see *Amniocentesis* on page 51) to detect Down syndrome. Potential heart abnormalities will be checked by a special ultrasound of the baby in the second trimester. Even if your partner chooses first-trimester screening, she will need another blood test in the second trimester to screen the baby for problems with his/her spine and intestinal tract.

Since this is a new type of testing, it may not be available in your area or your physician may not be offering it routinely. Many physicians utilize another test, the Quad Screen, to screen the baby for Down syndrome, other common chromosome problems, and spinal and intestinal tract abnormalities (see *Prenatal Screening* on page 48). This blood test is performed between the sixteenth and twentieth week of pregnancy. It detects Down syndrome offspring with a similar degree of accuracy as the first-trimester testing. If you have an abnormal test, your provider will suggest an amniocentesis (see *Amniocentesis* on page 51) to detect Down syndrome. Speak with your provider about the availability and his/her policy regarding this test.

At the present time, first- and second-trimester testing arc comparable. The choice of which test to performed will be determined by you and your physician. Because these tests are meant to screen a large number of women fast and inexpensively, there are going to be some false-positive and negative test results. Despite their limitations, they detect the majority of affected babies.

The experts tell me that we are just at the beginning of a new era in prenatal screening. In the near future we will expand our testing and accuracy in detecting Down syndrome and other chromosomal affected babies. I expect that in the next edition of *Pickles*, I will have new information to share on this subject

OFFICE VISITS—A visit is scheduled every four weeks. At each visit your partner will be weighed, will have her blood pressure measured, and will provide a urine sample. The physician will check the baby's growth and try to hear the fetal heartbeat with a Doppler, a device designed to audibly pick up the heartbeat. Usually, the heartbeat can be heard after the tenth week. DON'T MISS THIS VISIT! Not only is hearing the heartbeat for the first time exciting, it also represents a significant reduction in the risk of miscarriage. The monthly visit is an opportunity to review the progress of the pregnancy, ask questions, and develop a relationship with the doctor.

She is asking about...

It is nine p.m., and your partner is dead tired. She is getting ready for bed and notices something weird. She looks around the room and hones in on you. Once eye contact is made, you know you are a dead duck. She is about to tell you one of those mysterious symptoms of early pregnancy. Most of the time, you wish she'd pick up the phone and call the doctor, but she won't. And you definitely don't want her calling her friends again. The last time she did that, it took you hours to calm her down.

This section deals with the most common concerns your partner may have during the first three months and helps you decide what is going on and when to call the doctor. Please be patient, listen with interest, and maintain your composure. We are just a phone call away!

ABDOMINAL PAIN—Early pregnancy is fraught with strange sensations—most often, cramps and assorted pains. Typically this is the result of the uterus growing. If you listen to your partner, you can distinguish between the various types of discomfort and reassure her.

Crampy pain—Diffuse, low stomach cramps involving the entire pelvic region. This pain is frequently associated with constipation. It comes in waves of increasing intensity and diminishes after a bowel movement.

Menstrual cramps—Mild discomfort reminiscent of menstrual cramps noted around the pubic bone. These cramps occur as the uterus expands. Many women panic when they feel these pains, expecting their period to start any minute. Don't worry! This is a sign of a growing baby.

Persistent, intense cramping around the pubic bone, associated with vaginal spotting or bleeding, should be reported immediately to the doctor. This may be a sign of an impending miscarriage.

Sharp pain—Stabbing, sharp pain on either side of the low pelvis. The enlarging uterus pulling on its supporting ligaments usually causes this discomfort.

You should contact the doctor if your partner has persistent, severe abdominal pain. This may represent an ovarian cyst or a pregnancy in the fallopian tube, also known as an ectopic pregnancy.

Tugging pain—Pulling and tugging on either side of the low pelvis. This discomfort is in response to the stretching of the ligaments that support the growing uterus. The pain is intermittent and can be reduced by changing position, such as lying on the opposite side.

Anytime abdominal pain is severe and persistent, contact the doctor immediately!

ALCOHOL—We strongly discourage any alcohol consumption during pregnancy. Drinking can cause a serious birth condition called fetal alcohol syndrome.

BACK PAIN—Hormones released early in pregnancy may loosen the back and cause low back pain. Jobs requiring bending, twisting, prolonged standing, or lifting may trigger back pain. Sitting at a desk or driving a car may also lead to a backache. Using proper body mechanics will help reduce the discomfort. In some cases, the pain can become quite severe and may require a consultation with an orthopedic surgeon.

You will win brownie points and her admiration if you give her a back rub, ice her back, or offer her a heating pad. Some of my patients utilize a massage therapist with specialized training in pregnancy massage. It is a better gift than roses!

BLOATING—The hormones of pregnancy do a job on the intestinal tract, especially in the beginning. In addition to nausea and constipation, women feel their stomach is puffy even before you can see the difference. Most assume the baby is growing, pushing the belly outward. They're mistaken. The baby is still very small. In reality, the hormones cause an intestinal slowdown, leading to an accumulation of fluid, gas, stool, and a puffy belly. The bloating tends to diminish as the uterus takes center stage.

BLURRY VISION—The eye shape may actually change during pregnancy, resulting in blurry vision. You can reassure your partner that her vision will improve once the pregnancy is over. Annoying visual changes should be evaluated by an ophthalmologist.

BREAST DISCHARGE—Clear or yellow fluid may leak from the breast. Although breast discharge is more common in the third trimester, it is also normal during early pregnancy. Breast discharge is quite common during foreplay too. Bloody discharge should be reported to a physician for further evaluation.

BREAST MASS—Surging hormone levels can cause the breast tissue to thicken. The obstetrician should evaluate abnormal areas carefully with surgical consultation, as needed. In selected cases, mammograms and breast biopsies may be necessary. Rarely is breast cancer detected during pregnancy.

BREAST TENDERNESS—Sore, swollen breasts are a common sign of a healthy pregnancy. The associated discomfort eases as the pregnancy progresses.

CAFFEINE—There is no reason to totally avoid caffeine while pregnant. In other parts of the world, many women drink caffeinated beverages, including coffee and tea, and have normal pregnancies. I advise my patients to moderate their intake of caffeine. Decaffeinated beverages are an excellent alternative.

CALCIUM—Daily calcium ingestion is essential to the baby's growth and development. The prenatal vitamins contain only a portion of the daily requirement of 1200 mg. Milk, cereal, yogurt, and cheese are good dietary sources of calcium. For those who don't consume enough calcium, supplements such as Tums are a good alternative. They are also an effective treatment for heartburn, a common concern later in the pregnancy. Check the label to figure out how many tablets are needed to meet her daily requirement.

If your partner is lactose intolerant, buy her calcium supplements and reassure her that the baby will do just fine.

CHICKEN POX—For women who have had chicken pox, exposure during pregnancy is safe. Avoid infected children if your partner is unsure of her immune status. If she is exposed to an infected child, she should have a blood test to check her immunity. A susceptible woman who has had close contact should receive treatment with immunoglobulin to reduce her risk of contracting chicken pox or reduce the severity if she becomes infected.

If your partner is not immune and contracts the disease during pregnancy, the consequences differ based upon when in the pregnancy she is exposed. Some of the concerns are listed below.

First-trimester infection—Increased risk of birth defects in the baby.

Second-trimester infection—Increased risk of pneumonia in the mother. Rare effect on the baby.

Third-trimester infection—Increased risk of pneumonia in the mother. Delivery should be avoided until all the pox have crusted. This helps reduce the risk of transmitting the virus to the baby after delivery. It also gives your partner time to build up her own immunoglobulins, which can be shared with the baby if she nurses.

If she delivers between five days before the onset of chicken pox or five days after it appears, the baby can be treated with a medication to help prevent the infection.

If your partner lives in a home where a child has active chicken pox when she delivers, I strongly recommend having the infected child stay with relatives or friends until the pox have crusted. You should speak with your partner's obstetrician or the child's pediatrician concerning their recommendations too.

CHICKEN POX VACCINE—I would not have a child in the family vaccinated or have your partner exposed to a child recently vaccinated during pregnancy if she is not immune. Although infection is rare, there have been scattered reports of women becoming infected from presumed contact with a vaccinated child.

Pregnant women should not receive the vaccine either.

CHORIONIC VILLUS SAMPLING (CVS)—A genetic test performed around the tenth week of pregnancy. The test may be appropriate for women with a high likelihood of delivering a child with a chromosomal abnormality based on her age or family history. As compared to an amniocentesis, CVS is done six weeks earlier and has a slightly higher risk—1 percent—of losing the pregnancy.

The test involves placing a small plastic tube into the uterus and removing some of the placental cells. The tissue is sent to a lab and grown. Seven to ten days later, the chromosomal results are generally available.

Women undergoing CVS must understand that the test results are limited to the chromosomes. Further blood testing with an alpha fetoprotein is needed in the second trimester to evaluate the baby's nervous and intestinal systems. A woman with an abnormal alpha fetoprotein is offered an amniocentesis (see *Amniocentesis* on page 51).

Despite its limitations, I suggest CVS for patients when both partners are carriers of a genetic disorder such as sickle-cell anemia or Tay-Sachs disease. I encourage CVS to my patients who are forty years of age or older due to their higher risk of having a chromosomal abnormal pregnancy.

COLDS AND FLU—Each doctor has his or her own unique set of treatment recommendations for colds and flu in early pregnancy. Consult your partner's physician about the use of over-the-counter preparations and antibiotics.

COLORING HAIR—There is no conclusive medical information as to whether exposure to the chemicals used in coloring hair can be harmful to the baby. Common sense dictates waiting until the second trimester to tinker with the hair. Why expose the baby during its most critical time to chemicals? Highlighting hair is a safe alternative, since there is limited contact between the coloring agent and the scalp. Tell your partner to forget about perms. They don't hold well during pregnancy.

CONSTIPATION—Pregnancy tends to slow the movement of food through the intestines. As a result, constipation becomes a real problem for many women. Eating food high in fiber, increasing fluid intake, or taking a fiber preparation such as Metamucil or Fibercon will help fight this pregnancy-long problem. Since pregnancy vitamins contain extra iron, which is a constipating agent, I will often switch patients to a regular vitamin to ease the problem.

CRAVINGS—Be prepared for those late-night runs to the supermarket. It might be for a healthy dose of pickles and ice cream or some other exotic food combination. No matter what your partner wants to eat, smile and enjoy the experience. Her body is doing its job, demanding nutrients to help grow a beautiful, healthy baby. I've seen ardent vegetarians become ravenous meat eaters and spicy-food fans turn into bland broiled-chicken-and-potato lovers. As long as my patients watch their weight and eat some protein, carbohydrates, and fats, I do not question their food choices. My motto is "If she wants it, let her eat it!" After the first trimester the cravings will subside for many women.

DENTAL VISITS—I encourage my patients to go ahead with their annual dental screening. Cleanings can be performed, but only emergency X rays should be done. A lead apron must be draped over your partner's abdomen prior to taking the X ray. This greatly reduces the radiation exposure to the baby. Make sure your partner informs the dental technician that she is pregnant. Patients may have cavities filled and root-canal work done during pregnancy. Your dentist and obstetrician should communicate regarding the type of anesthesia to be administered. During cleanings or after brushing their teeth, many women experience bleeding gums. This is very normal.

DIET/NUTRITION—You may notice your partner becoming very focused on the type of food she eats. Perhaps she is trying to eat a measured amount of vegetables, carbohydrates, and protein. You might even think she is going a little nuts. In reality, she is trying to deal with the loss of control. Strange changes are altering everything about her body, and she can't stop it. I believe women frequently fight back by regulating their food intake. If you think your partner is being a little too rigid in her diet, remind her that cavewomen managed to survive pregnancy without pregnancy cookbooks or a scale to weigh their food.

DRUGS—The use of illicit drugs is harmful to your baby. Babies exposed to drugs tend to be smaller, addicted at birth, and have learning difficulties. In addition, cocaine is linked to an increased number of fetal deaths.

ECTOPIC PREGNANCY—Pregnancy growing outside the uterus, usually in the fallopian tube. It occurs in one of every eighty pregnancies and is a life-threatening condition. Women with a history of infertility, pelvic infections, ectopic pregnancy, or abdominal surgery are at high risk.

The symptoms include vaginal bleeding and/or abdominal pain. The diagnosis is made with the aid of an ultrasound and blood tests for human chorionic gonadotropin—the pregnancy hormone. Unfortunately, there is no way to save the pregnancy when it is outside the uterus.

The condition requires surgical removal of the ectopic by laparoscopy or treatment with a special medication to dissolve the tubal pregnancy. Both are acceptable ways to treat the condition. The choice of treatment is based on the size of the ectopic pregnancy and risks of complications to your partner.

EXERCISE—Your partner should maintain her current level of exercise, keeping her pulse under 140 beats per minute. Biking, swimming, and walking tend to be the best exercises for pregnant women. Make sure your partner drinks adequate fluid during exercise. Women experiencing fatigue or morning sickness, especially in the first trimester, find it difficult to exercise. This is normal. When they feel better, exercise can be resumed.

As your partner's belly grows, abdominal crunches and other exercises that require her to lie flat on her back should be avoided. Not only do they add extra strain on the abdomen and back, they tend to make her feel light-headed as well.

FATIGUE—Many women are surprised by the extent of their early pregnancy fatigue. Going to bed early and waking up late do not ease the overwhelming exhaustion. There is nothing wrong with this feeling. The fatigue usually goes away by the end of the first trimester. If your partner is feeling frustrated by the exhaustion, remind her of the remarkable job she is doing along with her daily activity. She is making arms, legs, kidneys, etc. She's entitled to be tired. It sounds like hard work to me!

FETAL HEART SOUND—Near the end of the first trimester the baby's heart can be heard with a special instrument called a Doppler. The heart sounds like a steam engine chugging along or a rhythmic swishing. The normal range for the heart rate is between 120 to 160 beats per minute. In the first trimester the heart rate may creep up into the 170 range without being a source of alarm.

We understand the stress that is created when the heartbeat is not heard. For this reason, most obstetricians will not attempt to hear the fetal heartbeat until they feel there is a good chance of finding it, typically after the tenth week. Large-size women and cases where the uterus rests away from the abdominal wall make it more difficult to hear the fetal heartbeat. For these patients we more often will wait until twelve weeks to make an attempt to hear the heartbeat. In cases where the heartbeat is not heard, we will perform an ultrasound to check on the baby's health.

FLU VACCINE—The Centers for Disease Control recommends that every woman who will be pregnant during the influenza season should be vaccinated.

FISH—The Food and Drug Administration advises pregnant women to avoid eating swordfish, king mackerel, shark, or tilefish. These fish have been found to contain significant levels of mercury, which can cause problems for a baby. Other authorities suggest limiting consumption of tuna steaks to once every two weeks, canned Albacore (white) tuna, to one serving a week, or a maximum of two servings of light canned tuna per week.

HEADACHE—A common first-trimester complaint. Most women tend to suffer without calling their doctor. I understand their reluctance to take medication; however, acetaminophen is perfectly safe. Why should she endure the miscry? If the headache isn't relieved with medication, I suggest calling the physician's office.

KITTY LITTER—Cat owners take note. This is a hot issue. There is a potential infection called toxoplasmosis found in cat feces. It can be passed on to the baby if your partner inhales fumes from a litter box. This holds true only if your cat goes outdoors and eats wild animals. If your cat is exclusively an indoor animal, there is no issue. Incidentally, many cat owners are already immune, having been exposed to this mild infection in the past. They can't transmit toxoplasmosis to their baby.

This infection is another over-publicized hype. In reality, very few babies become infected, and even fewer will suffer repercussions from their in-the-womb exposure. If there is concern, a blood test can be ordered to check your partner's immune status. Routine screening is not recommended in the United States.

I have found that the best solution is for you to take over litter box duties for the duration of the pregnancy, rendering this a moot point.

LIFTING—Careful bending and lifting can be performed during pregnancy without injury. As pregnancy progresses, many women find it increasingly difficult to lift the same amount. Under no circumstance should your partner risk injury by lifting more than she is physically able. Please alert the physician if your partner's job requires unusual amounts of lifting or bending.

LIGHT-HEADEDNESS—Experiencing a feeling of passing out or seeing spots in front of one's eyes is a very common symptom throughout pregnancy. Early in pregnancy this symptom is often attributed to a lack of sugar in the blood (low blood sugar) or heart palpitations. Many of my patients experience light-headedness when they get up too fast or stand in a hot shower too long. Being aware of the cause can lead to an easy solution, such as eating more often, getting up slower, or moving one's feet while showering. There is nothing to worry about unless your partner experiences a blackout. In this specific case, call her physician.

LOSS OF URINE—The uterus presses down on the bladder throughout pregnancy. Standing up suddenly or sneezing may trigger a sudden loss of urine. To help prevent this annoyance, your partner can perform Kegel exercises.

> *Kegel exercises*—While your partner is urinating, have her try to stop her flow. Once she can accomplish this, have her practice tightening the muscles throughout the day with a goal of thirty repetitions in all. Many women forget to do the exercise, so I suggest that every time they use the telephone, they do one Kegel.

Despite the exercise, leaking can still occur. Your partner should consider wearing a mini-pad to stay dry.

MISCARRIAGE—The loss of the baby before viability. It doesn't matter if a miscarriage happens at six weeks or six months. A pregnancy failing to provide a healthy baby is a tragedy and should be treated with sensitivity and support. Unfortunately, upward of 40 percent of all conceptions end in a miscarriage. Most miscarriages happen (70 percent of the time) because the woman's body recognizes an imperfection in the embryo that would have prevented the baby from being healthy.

Although bleeding is the most common sign of an impending miscarriage, one may notice the end-of-pregnancy symptoms (nausea, bloating, fatigue, or sore breasts). Other times, the diagnosis is not made until an office visit between the tenth and twelfth weeks, when the physician fails to hear the baby's heartbeat. The doctor will order an ultrasound to confirm his/her suspicion.

If vaginal bleeding does occur, a phone call to a physician is the first order of business. The doctor will try to establish the cause of bleeding by talking with your partner. A physical exam will clarify the situation. For a pregnancy beyond six weeks, an ultrasound can be done to check for the baby's heart rate. With an earlier pregnancy, a series of blood tests performed over several days can establish the baby's health.

> *Ultrasound*—A technology that uses sound waves to help visualize the fetus. If the pregnancy is beyond six weeks, the baby's heartbeat can usually be seen. The absence of a heartbeat indicates a miscarriage.

> *Beta Human Chorionic Gonadotropin (B-HCG)*—A blood test best used in early pregnancy when ultrasound may not see the fetus or the heart beat. The test measures the amount of pregnancy hormone in your partner's blood. In most cases, the test needs to be repeated in two days. If the blood level is dropping, a miscarriage is diagnosed. If the blood level is increasing, the pregnancy may still be healthy and further monitoring is required. Once the values rise above a critical number, an ultrasound can be performed.

Not every case of bleeding leads to a miscarriage. I have seen women bleed heavily and still deliver a healthy baby. Report any concerns to your partner's doctor.

Treatment

The treatment will be based upon your partner's medical condition. If your partner is experiencing heavy vaginal bleeding, the physician may suggest a surgical procedure known as a dilatation and curettage to clear out the remaining pregnancy tissue and stop the bleeding.

For those needing surgery, it is usually done in an operating room under anesthesia. The procedure is quick and well tolerated. Afterward many women experience mild menstrual cramps and light vaginal bleeding. Ibuprofen and a hug are the best medicine to deal with the post-procedural pain. Expect your partner to be tired for twenty-four hours after the surgery.

Sometimes I diagnose a miscarriage without bleeding. Under this circumstance I determine the likelihood that my patient will bleed heavily. Those most likely to bleed are offered surgery. In cases where the pregnancy loss was very early or when an ultrasound indicates there is little tissue in the uterus, I may opt to do nothing other than monitor the patient. It is quite possible that she will cleanse the uterus on her own by having a moderately heavy menstruation. If she bleeds lightly, I'll continue to monitor, and advise her about signs of an uterine infection.

If your partner develops a fever, foul vaginal discharge, or severe abdominal pain after a miscarriage or dilatation and curettage, call her physician immediately. This may be the sign of an infection or a pregnancy in the fallopian tube (see *Ectopic pregnancy* on page 29).

The consequences

I ask my patient to schedule a follow-up visit within four weeks. No matter how much counseling I've done at the time of the miscarriage, many of my patients erroneously believe they did something wrong and harbor unfounded guilt. Going over what happened and reinforcing the facts go a long way toward closure. I also tell my patients:

Your body is scrutinizing an early pregnancy to make sure the baby is perfect. It doesn't want to waste time and energy carrying a child that won't survive after birth. By turning off the nutrition to a problem pregnancy, your body is protecting you.

The risk of another miscarriage is the same as if it had never happened before. I know you won't believe me, but this is the truth for those who experience up to two miscarriages in a row.

It's okay to be sad. You have suffered a loss.

Your next period will return within four to six weeks. It tends to be different from your usual period.

Once you have gotten your first period, you can try to conceive at your discretion.

Your feelings are often overlooked after a miscarriage. I encourage you to support your partner and let her know how you feel. I still remember the due date of the baby my wife and I lost. It's still a sad day, three healthy children later.

MEDICATION—Other than prenatal vitamins, speak to a physician about the use of medications during pregnancy. For those who have medical conditions it's important to treat the condition while pregnant. Your partner should not stop medication because she is pregnant!

NAUSEA—You thought your partner wasn't going to get sick. Typically, nausea doesn't strike until the sixth to seventh weeks and varies in degree. It should ease up between the twelfth and fourteenth weeks. Nausea can be categorized based on its symptoms.

> *Mild*—A constant sense of nausea that doesn't lead to vomiting. Many of my patients describe this as a continuously empty stomach. Eating food seems to help this feeling.

> *Moderate*—Episodes of nausea and vomiting. Eating food doesn't help reduce the nausea and may trigger bouts of vomiting. Vomiting doesn't happen each time she eats or drinks.

> *Severe (hyperemesis)*—Difficulty holding down food or fluid throughout the day. Your partner will have a difficult time working or even doing simple household tasks. Some signs of this extreme degree of morning sickness include chapped lips, a constant thirst, or reduced urination. This is a

good time to contact the doctor. While you are waiting for a return phone call, here are a couple of soothing thoughts.

Nausea is associated with a healthy pregnancy.

There are medications to help treat the symptoms.

Babies are very clever. They will get the nutrients they need from the mother even if she isn't eating.

In the end, your baby will be fine. My sister lost twenty-three pounds in the first few months and had a healthy daughter.

Treatments—Home Remedies

Separate liquids from solids by a half hour (i.e., no milk with cereal)

Avoid citrus (i.e., oranges, grapefruit, or their juices)

Eat bland food, such as toast or a bagel

Discontinue prenatal vitamins until feeling better

Drink flat soda

Ginger pills, 500 mg four times daily

Vitamin-B6 pills, 25 mg three times daily

Sea bands or Reliefbands for the wrist

Treatments—Medical

Your partner's doctor will evaluate her need for medical treatment.

Intravenous fluids at home or in an outpatient setting

Antinausea medications

Hospitalization

Please remember that nausea eases up as the pregnancy progresses. Even the worst case usually gets better over time. As long as your partner is receiving fluids, the baby will do just fine.

NUTRASWEET—There is no reason to avoid Nutrasweet. Although there are no studies regarding this sugar substitute, moderate intake is safe.

NUTRITION—Much has been written about eating during pregnancy. This is also one of the most overrated issues. If your partner is either overweight or underweight, her physician should make specific nutritional recommendations. For average-weight women, I suggest that they listen to their body. It has served them well up to this point, so why stop now? A well-balanced diet and prenatal vitamins including folic acid are sufficient to ensure a healthy pregnancy. It is a good idea to encourage your partner to avoid junk food and excessive desserts. As for pickles and ice cream or other cravings, go with the flow and be amazed.

PALPITATIONS—A skipping or racing heartbeat can happen. It's triggered by an increase in the amount of water in your partner's blood stream. This fluid is necessary to nourish the baby. Palpitations can be extremely annoying but aren't treated unless they lead to fainting episodes.

PHYSICAL CHANGES IN EARLY PREGNANCY—Common symptoms include bloating, sore breasts, low abdominal cramping, menstrual cramping, backache, and fatigue.

Just about every pregnant woman experiences pelvic cramping. When this happens, she's sure the pregnancy test was wrong and her period is coming. Don't worry. Cramping is a natural response as the uterus stretches.

SEX—There are lots of rumors about your partner's sexual interest. Some say her sex drive increases, and others say the opposite. As you will learn during this nine-month experience, listening to others will only confuse you more. Each couple is different. If your partner's libido is increased, great! If it is reduced, understand that it isn't you. She is expending her energy making that healthy baby.

SHORTNESS OF BREATH—This sensation can happen during exercise, walking, or at rest, and it is commonly referred to as air hunger. Your partner feels the need to take a big sigh here and there to catch her breath. There is nothing wrong with her. She isn't out of shape. It's another normal response to the hormones of pregnancy.

SHINGLES—If your partner has shingles, it won't pass to the baby. If your partner is exposed to a person with shingles and had had chicken pox in past, then she is perfectly safe.

If she has not had chicken pox, she has a small chance of becoming infected. Speak with her doctor. In this case it is a good idea to avoid spending time with people with active shingles.

SKIN CHANGES—Some women develop a slight darkening of the skin across the bridge of their nose and around their eyes. This benign condition is known as the mask of pregnancy. Others notice a line of dark tissue developing on their abdomen, which seems to split it in half. This is called the linea nigra, and it is also a harmless skin change. Both skin alterations resolve after delivery.

Acne can become an annoyance during pregnancy. Treating the skin with over-the-counter medication is frowned upon. Instead, clean the skin with soap on a frequent basis, or speak with a physician about topical antibiotic ointments.

Small growths called skin tags tend to pop up on the neck and chest. They are benign and do not require treatment during pregnancy. If your partner notices a change in a mole (color or growth), it should be evaluated by a physician.

SMOKING—Cigarette and cigar smoking are hazardous to pregnancy. Either can lead to poor growth or premature delivery of the baby. If your partner smokes, encourage her to quit. Each time your partner lights up, the baby is exposed to nicotine, carbon monoxide, and other hazardous chemicals. If she can't stop smoking, help her! If you smoke, lead by example. She'll find it easier to quit with your support. Speak to the physician about ways to help her stop smoking.

With fatherhood rapidly approaching, it's time for you to think about your future. Giving up smoking is the first gift to your newborn. We all know nonsmokers live healthier and longer, letting you enjoy fatherhood for many more years. Removing smoke from the home environment will improve your newborn's health too.

STRESS—Stress is not dangerous to a pregnancy unless your partner becomes ill or unable to eat due to the stress. Corrective steps need to be taken in this rare circumstance. Speak with the physician if you have specific concerns.

THIRST—Many of my patients notice an increase thirst. This is perfectly normal. It's caused by the body's increasing demand for fluid to help nourish the growing baby. No matter how much fluid your partner consumes, she isn't drinking too much.

TRAVEL—In an uncomplicated pregnancy there are no restrictions on travel, including airplane flights, through the second trimester. Even the metal detectors are safe! After the seventh month, travel restrictions may be suggested by the physician. Speak with your partner's doctor about her/his policy.

VAGINAL BLEEDING—One of the most common calls received by doctors pertains to vaginal bleeding, especially early in pregnancy. From brown staining to bright red vaginal bleeding, the amount and scope of blood vary widely, as does the ultimate outcome. Miscarriage is the most feared complication associated with bleeding. However, there are many instances of early pregnancy bleeding that do not represent a pregnancy loss.

The most common cause of bleeding is the implanting placenta trying to root itself in the uterus. This is a critical step in providing the baby with adequate nourishment. The placenta is digging into the uterus, searching for a blood supply to feed the growing embryo. Sometimes, blood is released during this process. Other times, bleeding can happen after a pelvic exam or sexual intercourse. This type of bleeding is not dangerous to the fetus. Regardless of your suspicion, vaginal bleeding merits a phone call to the physician.

VAGINAL INFECTION—It is uncommon for women to experience vaginal infections in early pregnancy. For those suffering a mild to moderate irritation, topical over-the-counter medications can be used safely. Occasionally the irritation is severe enough to justify a doctor's visit. In this case, don't hesitate to call.

WEIGHT GAIN—Expect your partner to gain between twenty and thirty-five pounds during the pregnancy. In the first trimester women gain less weight than in the subsequent trimesters. You shouldn't be worried if your partner doesn't gain much weight early in pregnancy.

Women experiencing mild nausea find eating a good way to control the sensation. They may gain weight rapidly. Once the nausea abates, the weight gain will balance out. Unfortunately, they may gain a few more pounds than their peers.

The monthly office visit is a good time to discuss weight gain and necessary dietary modification. For those having a problem, get on a scale weekly. If the weight keeps piling on, contact the physician. I will refer patients to a dietitian to help adjust their eating habits. It's important to get a handle on weight management early. Excessive weight gain can cause obstetrical complications.

In my experience, the father-to-be tends to gain weight during pregnancy. I am not sure if it is due to nerves, watching your partner continue to expand, or your trying to keep up with your partner's eating habits at the dinner table. Don't be surprised if you add ten pounds along the way.

SECOND TRIMESTER

Welcome to the second trimester. You have survived your partner's overwhelming fatigue, irritability, and strange eating habits. Now she is acting more like the woman you love and cherish. And you are getting used to the fatherhood idea and are thinking about baseball bats, gloves, and your child's first home run. Maybe you can even see yourself outside chasing a soccer ball and teaching your little one a move you learned in high school.

The second trimester is the best part of the pregnancy. Your partner is feeling better. Overnight, her stomach has popped out, and maternity clothes are occupying the closet. Just when you get used to her new figure, she will sprout again. Along the way the fetus will turn into a real person, kicking and moving around while you watch in amazement.

As you make the transition into your role as a parent, you'll have many financial responsibilities. However, there's one important responsibility that my not be as apparent as others. It involves ensuring future economic security for your child and your partner. Many of us forget about protecting our family by purchasing life and disability insurance, but these are important considerations for everybody's sake. Please take the time to consider providing this coverage for your family. The start of the second trimester is a good time to take this step.

Get ready for some fun and some important decisions.

TERMS TO KNOW

First, the new vocabulary words:

Alpha fetoprotein (al-fa fee-toe-pro-teen)—A protein secreted from the baby that can be detected in the mother's blood. The level can predict the risk of nervous system and intestinal disorders.

Amniocentesis (am-nee-o-cen-tee-sis)—A procedure during which fluid is removed from the sac around the fetus. The fluid is then sent for alpha fetoprotein and chromosome testing.

Amniotic fluid—Clear liquid surrounding the fetus.

Amniotic sac—Bag composed of two tough layers that hold the fetus and amniotic fluid.

Chromosome (crow-moe-so-m)—The structure that holds the genetic material that guides the development of a fetus. Humans have forty-six chromosomes (twenty-three pairs). An XX chromosome indicates a female, and an XY indicates a male. Chromosomal abnormalities may be associated with birth defects ranging from mild to severe.

Neural tube defect—A variety of defects of the nervous system from the brain to the spine. The most common type is spina bifida.

Spina bifida—A condition occurring in two out of every one thousand births in the United States, unrelated to the woman's age. In this condition the fetal spine fails to develop properly, leaving a hole in the spine. Paralysis below the damaged spot leads to significant medical problems throughout life.

Quad screen blood test—Four blood tests that help screen for chromosome, neural tube, and intestinal disorders.

OFFICE VISITS—Second-trimester office visits occur monthly. Your partner's blood pressure, weight, and urine will be checked at each appointment. The doctor will measure the baby's growth and listen to its heart. By the twentieth week your partner's stomach will be measured from the top of her pubic bone to the top of her uterus. This number is recorded in centimeters and used to make comparisons of the baby's growth from visit to visit. One great thing about the metric system in obstetrics is that

the measurement of the uterine size in centimeters corre-
lates closely with the number of weeks your partner is
pregnant. For example, if the uterus measures 22 cm,
we'd estimate your partner is around 22 weeks pregnant.

An early second-trimester office visit should include a
discussion about the upcoming prenatal screening, which
includes a quad-screen blood test and an ultrasound. For
women age thirty-five or older at the time of the expected
birth or those with certain genetic histories, an amniocentesis is recommended.

Prenatal screening

The biggest obstacle to enjoying the second trimester is
the *quad-screen blood test* offered between the fifteenth
and twentieth weeks of pregnancy to help determine the
health of the baby. Because the test is meant to screen a
large number of women fast and inexpensively, there are
going to be some false-positive and negative test results.
Despite its limitations, the test picks up the majority of
babies with chromosome and neural-tube defects.

In the following section I will explain the components
of the quad screen.

PART 1

ALPHA FETOPROTEIN (AFP)—A component of the
quad-screen blood test used to detect the risk of neural-

tube defects, including spina bifida and several intestinal disorders.

Normal alpha fetoprotein—The baby has a very small chance of having a neural-tube defect or certain gastrointestinal disorders.

Elevated alpha fetoprotein level—If the test shows an abnormally high level, don't freak out. There are many reasons for an elevated level, such as twins, an incorrect due date, or a false-positive result. The physician will repeat the test before proceeding.

While waiting for the repeat test results to come back, remember what I said earlier. This is a screening test. Inevitably, there will be some false-positive results. In fact, 5 percent of all tests are abnormal the first time. By doing a little math, I can tell you that if your first test is abnormal, the chances of your having a normal baby are still 96 percent.

SECOND TEST RESULTS:

Normal—All is well and so is the baby.

Elevated—Perform an ultrasound to look at the baby in more detail and consider an amniocentesis (see *Amniocentesis* on page 51).

PART 2

QUAD SCREEN—A series of four blood tests that includes the alpha fetoprotein, HCG, estradiol, and inhibin A that is used to predict the risk of the baby having a chromosomal abnormality. As an example, the test may indicate a 1/1000 or 1/10 risk of having a specific chromosomal problem. If the test results are abnormal, indicating a risk greater than 1/270 of having a chromosome problem, the physician will suggest an ultrasound followed by an amniocentesis (see *Amniocentesis* on page 51). In this circumstance, repeating the quad screen is not an appropriate option.

ULTRASOUND—A radiology test using sound waves to create an image of the fetus. The test looks carefully at the baby from head to toe. Ultrasound is optimally performed around eighteen to twenty weeks and includes an evaluation of the heart, kidneys, stomach, intestines, brain, spine, and extremities. In many cases, the sex of the baby can be determined. Although ultrasound may miss small abnormalities, it should pick up the most important problems. Any unusual findings should be discussed with your partner's obstetrician.

An ultrasound also determines the number of babies, location of the placenta, amount of amniotic fluid, and reconfirms the due date. One big misconception about the second-trimester ultrasound involves the due date. This scan is less accurate than a first-trimester ultrasound, a known last menstrual period, or an early visit to the doctor in predicting the due date. For people without an early evaluation, ultrasound is better than a guess, but it can be off by as much as two weeks!

For patients with abnormal blood testing, the ultrasound may offer some instant information. In the case of an *elevated AFP*, a careful evaluation of the fetal spine, head, and gastrointestinal tract can detect a problem. Although an amniocentesis is still necessary, we may determine the nature of the problem while waiting for the amniotic fluid AFP result, which usually takes a few days.

When an *abnormal quad screen* has occurred, a careful ultrasound may detect birth defects consistent with a chromosomal abnormality. From my experience, uncovering a chromosomal problem with ultrasound is rare. The definitive diagnosis will come from the results of the amniocentesis.

AMNIOCENTESIS—This test is offered to all women age thirty-five or older when the baby is born. Couples with a family history of a genetic disease, as well as those with an abnormal quad screen, are also candidates for the test. Before doing an amniocentesis, it's important to understand the risks associated with the procedure. They include the bag of water breaking and uterine infections. When either complication occurs, there is a strong chance of losing the baby. I tell patients that 1 out of every 200 amniocenteses will result in the loss of the pregnancy.

Procedure

After cleansing the stomach with an antiseptic solution, a slender needle is placed into the amniotic

sac under ultrasound guidance. Approximately 4 tea-
spoons of the amniotic fluid are removed and sent
for AFP and chromosomal analysis. The test takes
about one minute to perform.

Results—AFP

The AFP result is available in a few days.

A **normal** level is indicative of a baby without a
neural tube or certain gastrointestinal defects.

An **abnormally high** result prompts further testing from the fluid, including an acetylcholinesterase
and fetal hemoglobin level. Together the tests can
help determine if the baby has a significant health
problem. The fetal hemoglobin test comes back
quickly, whereas the acetylcholinesterase can take an
additional week to return. The test results should be
discussed with your doctor.

Results—Chromosomes

The test takes between seven and twenty-one days
to be completed. The long delay is due to the need
to grow the chromosomes in the laboratory. Once
grown, the chromosomes are counted many times to
verify the results.

A normal result is a source of great relief.
Although it doesn't guarantee a perfect baby, it does
exclude Down's syndrome and other conditions

associated with an abnormal number of chromosomes. If your partner had an amniocentesis due to an abnormal quad screen and the chromosomes are normal, you have just survived the worst episode of the pregnancy. You can relax and enjoy the next twenty weeks.

An **abnormal** result is a huge disappointment and a source of confusion. Although you may seek a second opinion, the chromosomal studies are extremely accurate. Speak to your partner's physician regarding the consequences of the test. The doctor may suggest counseling with a genetic specialist.

DOES THE AMNIOCENTESIS HURT?—An amniocentesis hurts about as much as getting your blood drawn. Your partner might notice an achy sensation at the site of the amniocentesis over the next few days.

SHOULD MY PARTNER REST AFTER HAVING AN AMNIOCENTESIS?—Although there is no medical research addressing this question, I suggest a reduced level of activity on the day of the amniocentesis. Your partner can work, but I wouldn't lift heavy furniture or go to an aerobics class until the next day.

After the test I encourage my couples to get a bite to eat. Both of you have just gone through a tension-filled experience and a tasty treat can help ease your collective stress.

She is asking about...

ABDOMINAL PAIN—Most women notice their expanding stomach rising up beyond their belly button by the midpoint of pregnancy. The growth triggers pulling pains on either side or around the navel. Your newly active baby can aggravate Mom with his/her movements or kicks, causing sharp pains across the belly. Most of the discomfort is mild and self-limiting. If the pain is severe and constant, check with your partner's physician.

BABY'S GROWTH—Around the fifth month the uterus pops. Your partner's stomach will become more obviously pregnant, and it's time for some serious maternity clothes. One of those innocent comments that will drive you crazy happens when she goes to buy her new wardrobe. Someone will look at her stomach and says, "You're too small. Something is wrong with your baby." Your partner will go bonkers! Be forewarned and armed with the following information. First-time mothers have strong stomach muscles, preventing the belly from protruding. This makes her stomach appear smaller than many expect. You should reassure her by saying, "Don't listen to them. Your doctor told you everything is going well. She/he is right. You are doing a great job!"

In subsequent pregnancies the story will be quite the opposite. People will be asking her if she's carrying twins. She'll nostalgically yearn for the days when people thought she was carrying small.

BATHING/SWIMMING—Both are safe throughout pregnancy regardless of any old wives' tale you have heard.

COXSACKIEVIRUS (HOOF-AND-MOUTH DISEASE)—A childhood illness more commonly seen in the summer. Most adults have already had the virus and won't get it again. If your partner experiences a rash and mouth ulcers, she probably has contracted the disease. The virus rarely causes serious problems for the mother or baby. Check with your partner's doctor if you have any questions.

EXERCISE—Exercising is a great idea. I have found women who exercise tend to gain less weight and have easier labors. Although your partner may not be able to keep up the same pace or routine as she did in the past, it is perfectly normal to modify her exercise program to suit her body's demands. Walking, biking, or swimming are all excellent ways to stay fit. Remind your partner to keep her pulse under 140 beats per minute, avoid exercising on her back, or performing abdominal crunches for the remainder of her pregnancy. Make sure she drinks adequate fluid while exercising and afterward.

FETAL MOVEMENT—Between sixteen and twenty-four weeks most women begin to feel the baby move. The sensation is described as gas, or butterflies in the stomach. After a few more weeks you might be able to feel the baby move if you rest a hand on your partner's uterus and wait patiently.

The movement pattern is quite unpredictable. There may be days when your partner doesn't recall feeling any baby movements. This is perfectly normal. Although there is a tendency to panic when this happens, tell your partner to relax. The baby is still quite small and may be moving, just not hard enough to let you know all is well, or perhaps your partner has been so busy with the rest of her life that she hasn't paid attention. In most cases, if you go about your normal activities, the baby will move again. If either of you is still concerned, have your partner eat something and sit down with a hand on her uterus. Wait an hour and see if she can feel any movements. The majority of babies will let her know everything is fine with a few swift kicks. If the baby still has not moved, you can call the physician.

If you contact my office, I will reassure your partner by scheduling an appointment to hear the heartbeat. Hearing that little thump-thump-thump is the best medicine to ease your anxiety.

Some texts suggest counting fetal movement as a way to monitor the baby's health. This is a good suggestion in the third trimester, not in the second. Speak with your partner's physician if you have any questions about the movement pattern.

FIFTH'S DISEASE—A common childhood illness caused by a virus that can be transmitted to a susceptible pregnant woman. Typically, I get a call from an expectant mother exposed to an infected child. I order a blood test to check if she is immune. If she has already had Fifth's Disease, she won't become infected.*

If she is not immune, I wait to see if she develops symptoms, which include sore throat, red rash, fever, joint aches, fatigue, and malaise. A follow-up blood test is performed in three weeks to see if she has contracted the illness.

Women who become infected need careful, frequent ultrasounds to monitor the baby. In the event that the baby shows signs of infection, the physician will make suggestions on further management. Even in this group, 95 percent of the children are born healthy.

GLUCOSE TESTING, ONE HOUR—Between the twenty-fourth to twenty-eighth weeks of pregnancy, a sugar-screening test is performed in the office, a lab, or hospital to detect the 3 percent of pregnant women who have pregnancy-induced diabetes. This test does not require your partner to fast in advance. All she has to do is drink a sweet orange or lime drink with a prescribed amount of sugar. One hour later her blood will be drawn.

Results:

> *Normal*—No diabetes. *Bon appetit.*

> *Elevated*—An elevated one-hour test doesn't mean your partner has diabetes. She needs a more definitive test, the three-hour glucose-tolerance test.

---

*Fifty percent of adults have already had Fifth's Disease and won't get it again.

GLUCOSE TESTING, THREE HOUR—A series of blood tests to diagnosis diabetes. After drawing a fasting blood sample, the woman drinks a prescribed amount of a sugar drink. Over the next three hours her blood is sampled hourly. If two or more of the blood tests are elevated, she has pregnancy-induced diabetes.

The treatment depends on the test results. Most women are placed on a special diet to limit the amount of sugar they eat. Thereafter, their glucose levels are monitored with blood tests or home glucose-monitoring devices. In rare cases she will need to take shots of insulin to control her sugar level. Speak with your partner's physician for more information on this test and the management of diabetes in pregnancy.

Diabetic diets aren't so bad. They cut out some of the goodies, but there is plenty of food to eat. Following the doctor's dietary suggestions will help ensure a healthy pregnancy and keep the baby from growing too large.

HEARTBURN—Burning in the mid-chest and/or an acid taste in the throat between meals are the most common complaints. Your partner can reduce this annoyance by eating small, frequent meals, avoiding food in the later evening, and sleeping on several pillows. Antacids such as calcium-rich Tums, Mylanta, or Maalox help to ease the symptoms. Over-the-counter Zantac and Tagamet have been studied during pregnancy and can be taken for unremitting heartburn. If the discomfort persists, speak with the doctor.

HOT TUBS/JACUZZI—We want to avoid exposing the embryo or fetus to heat because it may have some negative effect on the baby. By sitting in a hot tub or hot Jacuzzi, the baby is placed in an unhappy environment. Why not turn the thermostat down, keeping it under 98 degrees at all times, and enjoy a warm hot tub or Jacuzzi instead?

LIGHT-HEADEDNESS—Your partner may feel as if she is going to pass out, or she may see spots in front of her eyes. These are common symptoms throughout pregnancy. In the midst of pregnancy this is more typically caused by a rapid heart rate, or as the result of lying on one's back or waiting too long to eat. Standing up too fast or standing in a hot shower commonly triggers light-headedness in many patients too. Being aware of the cause can lead to an easy solution, such as eating more often or getting up slower. If your partner passes out or the episodes persist, contact her doctor.

LYING ON THE BACK—Since most pregnancy books advise women to avoid lying on their back throughout pregnancy, you can only imagine the frantic phone call I receive when a patient discovers that she slept on her back.

After calming her down, I explain the facts surrounding this myth. When a pregnant woman lies on her back, the uterus may press on the large blood vessels carrying blood from her legs and pelvis, slowing its return to the heart. The fear is that this supposedly reduces the amount of blood available to the baby. Perhaps this is true in a rare case, but nobody has ever proved that it is dangerous to the baby.

I reassure my patients by telling them that the baby is perfectly safe and has not suffered any injury. I continue by explaining one of the great truths of pregnancy. God was smart enough to create woman so she'd turn on her side, awake or asleep, to improve her circulation in this situation. If your partner is still worried, remind her that cavewomen managed to have babies without prepared childbirth classes or maternity books. Sometimes we have to trust our body to do the right thing.

To answer the question simply: Your partner should sleep any way she feels comfortable.

There is one exception to this rule. She should avoid lying on her back while exercising.

NUTRITION—Encourage your partner to eat healthy. By now many of the cravings have vanished, and her appetite has increased. This is a good time to check the total weight gain and make adjustments if she has been gaining more than a pound per week (i.e., 22 weeks equals 22 pounds).

RH INCOMPATIBILITY—Each of us has a blood type: A, B, AB, or O and a Rh positive or negative. When a baby is conceived, it will have its own blood type and Rh coming from you and your partner. If your partner has Rh-negative blood and you have Rh-positive blood, there is a chance that she will develop antibodies against the baby's blood cells (if the baby is positive). The first pregnancy is unaffected. Subsequent pregnancies are a different story. They are at an increased risk of serious complications for the baby.

Rh disease has been virtually eliminated by giving an injection of the medication Rhogam at twenty-eight weeks of pregnancy to Rh-negative women. Rh-negative women having an amniocentesis should be given Rhogam at the time of the test and an additional dose at twenty-eight weeks of pregnancy.

At delivery the baby's Rh status will be determined. If the baby is Rh negative, Rhogam is not necessary. Mothers of Rh-positive offspring need another shot of Rhogam.

Rhogam may also be given to an Rh-negative woman if she has early pregnancy bleeding, a miscarriage, or if the pregnancy continues more than thirteen weeks since the twenty-eight-week Rhogam injection.

In the rare case that a woman is found to be Rh sensitized, she should be referred to a specialist for further management. Although these pregnancies may be complicated, they often result in the birth of a healthy baby.

If both parents are Rh negative, the baby will not be affected by Rh disease.

TRAVEL—Leisure travel should be completed by the end of the second trimester, assuming the pregnancy has been healthy. For those who desire to travel in the third trimester, speak with the physician about her/his policy.

While traveling, I recommend that my patients get up and walk around every few hours. This will reduce the risk of blood clots developing in her legs.

VAGINAL BLEEDING—Most of the phone calls I get about bleeding in the second trimester are related to intercourse. In these cases I reassure my patient that the baby is just fine and that she should expect red or brown spotting for the next week. Slight spotting without intercourse warrants careful monitoring. If it persists or she experiences heavy or bright red, continuous vaginal bleeding, contact the physician immediately.

VAGINAL DISCHARGE—Changes in the hormone levels allow different bacteria to grow in the vagina. This increases the amount of secretion. Although the discharge is annoying, it rarely causes itching or odor. Most women wear a light pad to absorb the discharge. Foul-smelling discharge is unusual and should prompt a conversation with the physician.

If the discharge creates an itch, topical medication such as over-the-counter hydrocortisone cream can be applied sparingly.

THIRD TRIMESTER

By now your partner is into maternity clothes and sporting a more rotund shape. Colleagues and strangers are beginning to touch her belly as if it were some mystical Buddha, and they offer unsolicited pregnancy war stories and advice. Of course, nobody tells your partner about their easy birth experience, just the horror stories. If you don't get a few panicked calls after she's been tormented, you are one of the fortunate few.

On the baby front, your child is growing by leaps and bounds. Already two pounds, the baby has made a remarkable journey from embryo to fetus to your son or daughter-to-be. Keeping the baby in the uterus is the number one objective of the early third trimester. Any questions or problems should be discussed in depth with your partner's physician.

TERMS TO KNOW

Here is the third trimester lingo:

Breech—The baby is turned, so the buttocks or feet are closest to the birth canal.

Cesarean section—Abdominal delivery of the baby.

Contraction—Tightening of the uterus.

Dilatation—The diameter of the cervical opening.

Effacement—The thickness of the cervix.

Engaged—The fetal head is settled deep in the pelvis.

Epidural—A procedure in which a plastic tube is placed in the outer back and injected with numbing medication to relieve pain during labor.

Episiotomy (e-pee-zee-ah-toe-me)—Incision cut at the bottom of the opening of the vagina to create more space for the baby to come out.

Forceps—Metal instruments used to help deliver the baby vaginally.

Labor—Contractions that lead to the delivery of the baby. Dilatation and effacement of the cervix, as well as movement of the baby down the birth canal, are the hallmarks of this event.

Lamaze—A technique utilizing breathing and relaxation to deal with labor discomfort.

Position—The way the baby is facing in the pelvis.

Prepared childbirth—Classes that present information on pregnancy, labor, and delivery.

Station—The location of the baby's head in the woman's pelvis.

Vacuum—A soft plastic cup used to help deliver the baby vaginally.

OFFICE VISITS—Beginning in the third trimester, doctor's appointments will be more frequent. By the last month, visits will be weekly. The physician will monitor your partner's blood pressure, urine, and weight. In addition, the doctor will measure her uterus to check the baby's growth and position (head down, breech, or transverse lie), ask about the baby's movement pattern, and any unusual symptoms that your partner may be experiencing.

Many physicians start doing vaginal exams in the last month of pregnancy. This evaluation checks the cervix and its readiness for labor, the size of your partner's pelvis, and the baby's head position. Sometimes your partner will experience light cramping or bleeding after an exam. This is normal.

The pelvic exam reveals information on the effacement, dilatation, and station.

> *Effacement*—The cervix spends nine months holding the baby inside. Now it's time to let the baby out. In order to accomplish this goal, the cervix makes some major changes. To illustrate my point, I like to describe the cervix as a clenched fist ready to open up. Start at the baby finger and slowly peel the fingers away until only the thumb and index finger are touching. Have you noticed how thin the fist has become? This is analogous to the cervix thinning 100 percent. If you do an exam prior to all the fingers being unclenched, you have a percentage of the fist still present. This ranges between 0 and 100 percent. This is the same way we describe the effacement of the cervix.

In my opinion, effacement is the most important part of the exam. Thinning the cervix is the longest and most tedious part of labor. If your partner is 70 percent or more effaced, it bodes well for an easier labor.

> *Dilatation*—The cervix has to stretch open to let the baby pass into the birth canal. The measurements change from 0 to 10 centimeters (cm). Once the cervix has dilated to 10 cm, delivery is coming soon.

> *Station*—The baby must move out of the pelvis and through the birth canal to be delivered. The location of the head in relationship to the middle of

the pelvis is referred to as the station. The numbers go from -4 (head floating in the pelvis) to +4 (head coming out of the vagina).

Examples:

A patient with the following exam would be unlikely to go into labor soon.

0 percent effaced, 0 cm dilated, and –3 station.

A patient with the following exam would be likely to go into labor soon.

100 percent effaced, 3 cm dilated, and 0 station.

PELVIC SIZE—During a vaginal exam the doctor can get a sense of the size of the pelvis. This evaluation can help predict the likelihood of the baby fitting through the birth canal.

There are three different results.

Constricted pelvis means the bones are too narrow to let a normal-sized baby pass through the birth canal.

Borderline pelvis indicates the bones are tight but may allow for a vaginal birth of a normal-sized baby.

Adequate pelvis suggests the bones are far enough apart to allow for a vaginal delivery of a normal-sized baby.

THIRD TRIMESTER

The doctor's opinion as to the size of the pelvis has to be tempered by the likely size of the baby. For instance, a large baby can have a difficult time fitting through an adequate pelvis, whereas a small baby might squeeze through a constricted pelvis. In the end, estimating the size and shape of the pelvis isn't an exact science. The ultimate test is a "trial of labor" to see what happens.

BEFORE-DELIVERY PHYSICIAN RESPONSIBILITIES—A positive relationship should be well established between your family and the obstetrician. An open line of communication is critical to ensure the best outcome. *Never* feel intimidated about calling the doctor. We can't help unless we know what is going on. Don't do us any favors by not calling. In reality, it will make our job harder. If we can identify a problem early, the solution may be quite simple. Waiting too long might lead to the premature delivery of your baby! If there are any problems talking with the doctor or the office staff, now is the time to get things in order.

The doctor should review the following with you and your partner:

> What hospital she will deliver at
>
> Where to go in the hospital
>
> How to contact the office during and after hours
>
> When to call in labor
>
> What to do if the water breaks
>
> Management of labor pain
>
> Labor and delivery procedures
>
> Your birth options

HOSPITAL CHECKLIST—Packing the suitcase is a sobering time for an expectant couple. The reality is sinking in. Months of staring at your partner, wondering if she was really pregnant or just becoming a permanent beach ball have been answered. You are going to be a father soon. It's a good idea to have everything ready for your visit to the hospital. No need to panic as you try to find the essentials.

Here is a list of the items to bring:

Toothbrush/toothpaste/mouthwash

Brush/comb

Shampoo/conditioner

Deodorant

Makeup

Comfortable maternity outfit to wear home

Phone calling card

List of important phone numbers

Camera with flash, extra film, and batteries

Video camera (check the physician's policy and that of the hospital)/tripod

Bathrobe

Slippers

Nightgown or pajamas (not one of her best)

Light reading material (books or magazines)

Lollipops or hard sucking candy for your partner during early labor (check the physician's policy and that of hospital about these treats)

Snack food (in case the cafeteria is closed) for you

Items needed to prepare for your new baby's arrival:

Infant car seat

Crib and bedding

Bassinet and bedding

Diapers

Vaseline or A+D ointment

Alcohol and Q-tips

Onesies and newborn outfit

Infant nail clipper .

Baby shampoo

Pediatrician's phone number

Gentle baby detergent

Pacifier

Bibs

Bottles/formula

PREPARED CHILDBIRTH CLASSES—A MUST FOR FIRST-TIME PARENTS. No matter what type of birth experience you are planning, learning about childbirth and the facility where you'll be delivering is invaluable. The stress level decreases when you are aware of the various options for labor management. I guarantee that your partner expects you to be her support through these last weeks of pregnancy and delivery. The classes clue you in on what is going to happen and reinforce your important role.

Prepared childbirth is intended to educate you and your partner about the third trimester of pregnancy and birth options. These classes are not the same as Lamaze or Bradley courses, which teach different approaches to handling labor and delivery. Instead, prepared childbirth classes offer factual information on the physical changes associated with pregnancy, the process of childbirth, and ways to deal with labor pains. Most classes orient you to the birth hospital, as well as to their anesthesia policy during labor.

CHOOSING A PEDIATRICIAN/FAMILY PHYSICIAN— Picking a good doctor to care for your newborn will ease the fear of parenthood. A friendly, helpful voice giving counseling and advice is the key to a smooth transition into your new role. Asking friends and family is a great way to develop a list of doctors to consider. Don't forget to check with your partner's obstetrician. She/he will know all the area pediatricians/family doctors and is a great resource. Once you have your final list, call the doctor's office and ask some basic questions.

Is the doctor board certified in pediatrics or family medicine?

How many doctors are in the group?

Does the office have a separate area for sick children?

Does the office have evening and weekend hours?

What happens if my child gets sick on the weekend or during off-hours?

What hospital is the doctor affiliated with? (It is reassuring for your new pediatrician to see the baby in the hospital.)

Use the telephone interview as another way to evaluate the office. Was the receptionist pleasant and helpful? Did he/she seem knowledgeable? Remember, you're going to be relying upon these professionals for information and access to the physician.

Once you've made your decision, relax. You will meet the doctor in the hospital after delivery. Most likely, these daily visits will reinforce the wisdom of your choice. If not, you can always change doctors. Be patient. You'll find a good one.

She is asking about...

ABDOMINAL PAIN—A variety of abdominal pains become commonplace as the pregnant uterus grows.

Severe pain—Constant, severe pain is abnormal. The problem must be evaluated promptly. Contact your partner's doctor. Delay in diagnosis can have a negative impact on the mom and the baby.

Crampy stomach pains—Tightening of the uterus causes crampy mid-stomach pains. The discomfort lasts seconds to minutes and is often cyclic (comes and goes). They are known as Braxton-Hicks contractions. They are a sample of the type of contractions associated with labor. Don't start timing the pains unless the frequency is ten minutes apart, length is thirty seconds or longer, and intensity is increasing over time.

Sharp pains/dull aching—The baby can constantly press on a certain spot, irritating the muscles or nerves. The pressure causes a searing knifelike pain, a bruised sensation, or numbness. Usually you can feel the baby right beneath the tender spot. Your partner can try lying on the opposite side to coax the baby into another position.

Pulling pains—Tugging on either side that radiates into the groin is characteristic of ligament pain. Remember that the ligaments hold the uterus in place. As the uterus swings from side to side, the ligaments stretch, causing pulling pain. Switching positions may alleviate this discomfort.

BABY POSITION—Many women ask where the baby's head is located early in the third trimester. Although I am happy to answer the question, I preface my response by telling them the position is irrelevant. The baby will switch positions many times before labor.

In the last month of pregnancy the doctor will determine the head position. After an office visit you might receive a frantic phone call from your partner telling you the baby is "butt" first or feet first, also known as a breech. Don't panic. Three percent of all babies are breech at the end of pregnancy (see *Breech baby* on page 78).

BABY WEIGHT—Most patients want to know how big their baby is going to be when it is delivered. Generally, we can get a feel for the baby's size in the last several weeks. Although our estimate is just that, we are usually pretty accurate. The use of ultrasound to estimate the weight is no more accurate than our clinical judgment. In either case, we can be off by 10 to 15 percent.

BACK PAIN—Pregnancy can alter the way a woman stands, causing her to experience low-back discomfort. For others, the baby rests on the spinal nerves, creating a dull, throbbing, or a sharp, shooting discomfort that radiates into her leg or buttocks. Back pain can be reduced by wearing low-heel shoes and avoiding activities that make the back pain worse. Massage, ice packs, and warm heat are safe and helpful sources of relief. Modification of daily activities and work can help alleviate back pain. A visit to an orthopedic surgeon, physical therapist, or chiropractor may bring further relief. The use of a pregnancy belt may add additional support and comfort.

BATHING/SWIMMING—I can't tell you how many patients ask me if they can swim or bathe in the third trimester. The answer is a resounding yes! It's perfectly safe! Others ask me how they can determine if the bag of water has broken if they're in the water. I tell them that the amniotic fluid, which is 98 degrees Fahrenheit, is much warmer than bath or pool water. Also, the fluid will continue to leak after she dries off.

BLADDER INFECTIONS—An infection of the bladder can be difficult to diagnose during pregnancy. Bladder pressure and frequent urination are common throughout pregnancy and are also symptoms of a bladder infection. If burning happens with urination or the frequency of urination increases markedly, it's a good idea to speak with the doctor. She/he can evaluate a urine specimen for signs of infection. Early identification and treatment of a bladder infection will ease your partner's discomfort and reduce her risk of premature labor (associated with urinary infections).

BLOOD CLOTS—Painful red swelling in the leg can be caused by a blood clot, also known as phlebitis (flee-bye-tis). It's more common in the third trimester, after sitting for a long time or bumping one's leg. If you suspect your partner has a blood clot, contact the doctor immediately.

BLOOD DONATION—Most labs will not accept pregnant women as blood donors. Regardless of the reason, your partner shouldn't give blood. In rare circumstances family or friends may donate blood for your partner if they have a matching blood type. Please remember, it takes several days from the donation to the time the blood is available for use. The delay occurs because the blood must be carefully screened for a variety of infections that can be passed on to the recipient of the donation.

Most blood banks discourage you from donating blood for your partner. They feel that receiving your blood can trigger antibodies in your partner that could adversely affect future pregnancies.

THIRD TRIMESTER

BLOOD IN STOOL—A common complaint during all trimesters of pregnancy. Most often, rectal bleeding is caused by hemorrhoids. The amount of blood ranges from a small amount to a toilet full. Before beginning treatment, make sure the blood is coming from the rectal area. Placing a mini-pad in the underwear helps identify the location of the bleeding. Your partner should discuss the problem with her doctor.

BREAST DISCHARGE—A clear or yellow fluid often leaks from the breasts. Breast discharge is more common in the third trimester. It is normal and a sign of things to come. Bloody discharge should be reported to the physician.

BREAST MASS—Breast cancer is one of the most common malignancies of young women. It can be diagnosed during pregnancy. If an abnormal thickness or mass is discovered, please contact the doctor. Breast masses can be evaluated safely during pregnancy.

BREECH BABY—At delivery, only 3 percent of babies are in this unusual birth position where the baby's buttocks or feet are down in the birth canal, in front of the head. Envision the baby positioned with its head near your partner's ribs and its bottom or feet near her bottom. Confirmation of a breech presentation should be made with an ultrasound. Most breech babies are delivered by cesarean section. Under very limited circumstances, a breech baby can be delivered vaginally. Speak with your partner's doctor about this option.

There are several options available when you have a breech baby.

Option #1—Wait until thirty-seven weeks of pregnancy or beyond, confirm the baby is still breech, and perform an external cephalic version. If successful, wait for labor. If unsuccessful, schedule a cesarean section near the due date.

Option #2—Do nothing and reevaluate when your partner goes into labor. Some babies will turn spontaneously. You should have already discussed the type of delivery (vaginal or cesarean section) with the doctor.

Option #3—Schedule an elective cesarean section near the due date.

The baby can be turned around by the doctor. This is called external cephalic version (ECV).

ECV External Cephalic Version Procedure

The baby's heart rate is monitored and an ultrasound performed at the hospital prior to considering an ECV. If the baby has a good heart rate and there is a good amount of amniotic fluid surrounding the baby, the test can be considered. First an intravenous line is inserted into your partner's arm, and she is given medication to relax her uterus. Once the medication has taken effect, your doctor will place her/his hands on your partner's stomach, pressing down on the baby's head and buttocks at the same time. She/he will gently guide the baby into a somersault stopping

THIRD TRIMESTER

when the baby changes position and is now head down. Ultrasound is used throughout to monitor the progress of this brief procedure and the baby's heart rate.

ECV is successful 50 percent of the time. As with every procedure, there are risks associated with ECV. Speak with your partner's doctor about her/his experience with this procedure.

CARPAL TUNNEL SYNDROME (CTS)—An excessive fluid buildup in the wrist that irritates the nerve. It causes sharp pain, tingling, or numbness that radiates into the fingers, forearm, elbow, or shoulder. The pain is worse in the evening, after working on a computer or other jobs requiring repetitive use of the hand (i.e., dental hygiene). Prolonged nerve irritation can lead to muscle weakness and an inability to hold objects like a glass or pot. CTS can become annoying enough to wake your partner at night.

Treatment

Decrease the activity that triggers the pain

Soak the entire body in a luke-warm tub (reduces edema)

Wrist splints (available at surgical supply houses)

Consult with an orthopedic surgeon

Wrap the wrist with a bandage*

---

*Many of my patients prefer to use an inexpensive ACE bandage to ease their pain. I suggest that they loosely wrap the troublesome wrist in the same position that they'd maintain to shake hands. The wrap should restrict the wrist from bending easily but never be uncomfortable. The wrap can be used all day, or as needed.

Some women are plagued by CTS after delivery. They should keep using the remedies listed above. If the problem persists, visit an orthopedic/hand surgeon. CTS usually recurs with subsequent pregnancies.

CORD AROUND THE NECK—One of the worst days you may experience is if an ultrasound reveals that the cord is around the baby's neck. You will get a frantic call bringing you the news, along with everyone's terrible tale about this situation. For the remainder of the pregnancy your partner will be worried. I'm not suggesting that you dismiss her concerns; however, 15 percent of babies have done enough acrobatics to loop the cord around their neck! In almost all cases the baby does just fine. On rare occasions the baby can develop stress related to this condition. A heart-to-heart talk with the obstetrician will help alleviate her anxiety.

CORD-BLOOD COLLECTION—The placenta is rich in fetal blood cells. These cells can be stored as insurance against future illness (cancer) for the baby or a family member. Some of my patients choose to donate the cord blood to help cancer victims who are presently in need or for medical research.

For those couples choosing to collect the cells, it is important to order the collection kit and fill out the paperwork prior to your delivery. At the birth the obstetrician harvests the cells from the umbilical cord after clamping it. The sample is sent to the cord-blood company for storage. Please check with the obstetrician as to the availability of cord-blood collection in your community.

Cord-blood sampling is a hotly debated topic. There are questions as to the cost versus benefit, considering the small chance that your child or family will need the cells. Fortunately, the cost of cord-blood sampling is dropping rapidly, making it a more attractive option. As we speak, ground-breaking research is ongoing, and the future use of the cells may be substantial. Speak with your partner's physician about this option.

CONTRACTIONS—After the twentieth week your partner may notice bouts of uterine tightening. As long as the contractions are painless, there is no cause for alarm. Regular, painful contractions before the thirty-seventh week of pregnancy warrant a phone call to the doctor. This may be a sign of preterm labor (see *Preterm labor* on page 96).

DROPPING (LIGHTENING)—In the last few weeks of pregnancy your partner may notice a change in her stomach's shape or increased pelvic pressure. She'll comment on how much easier it is to breathe. At the same time, she'll say, "I feel the baby sitting between my legs." Don't panic. Don't call the doctor. The baby has moved deep into the pelvis in anticipation of labor. You don't have to put the bags in the car yet. Dropping can happen weeks before labor.

If the baby seems to have dropped months before your partner's due date, speak with the doctor.

EATING—Your partner's appetite begins to wane as her growing uterus exerts more pressure on her stomach. She will feel full faster. Don't worry. Encourage her to eat frequent small meals and drink plenty of fluid.

FALLING—Big, awkward, and even clumsy are accurate descriptions of a pregnant woman, especially later in pregnancy. As a result, falling is very common. Don't worry. The baby is surrounded by amniotic fluid. It makes for a great shock absorber and protects the baby. Falling on one's buttocks will not harm the baby. Falling directly on the stomach, on the side, or down the stairs is a different situation. Contact the doctor immediately. The doctor may want to monitor the baby in the office or hospital.

If your partner develops constant stomach pain or the baby doesn't seem to be moving the same after a fall, call the physician immediately.

FETAL GROWTH—As in the second trimester, the physician measures your partner's uterus from the pubic bone to the top of the uterus. The results (in centimeters) correlate with the number of weeks she's pregnant (i.e., 32 cm = 32 weeks pregnant). Large discrepancies, either too small or too big, alert the physician. In this situation an ultrasound will be performed to evaluate the baby's growth and the amount of fluid surrounding the baby (see *Ultrasound* on page 105).

FETAL MOVEMENT—My patients become accustomed to their baby's movement pattern in the last several months of pregnancy. It is a comforting sign that everything is all right. Obstetricians agree with this notion. Research has demonstrated that fetal movement is an important indicator of how he/she is doing. By the thirty-sixth week the baby should be moving *at least:*

TWO movements within an hour after each meal

or

TEN movements by noon

The baby's movement pattern changes in the last weeks of pregnancy. Subtle rolling, bumping, or kicking replaces the sharp kicks and stabbing sensations. These movements should all be counted.

If the baby doesn't move as I've suggested or its movements seem less than normal, CALL THE DOCTOR IMMEDIATELY. This may be a warning sign of a problem.

Often I get a phone call from a concerned couple asking about periods of hyperactivity in their baby. They are concerned that the baby is gasping for breath or in distress. I calm their fears and tell them, "A moving baby is a healthy baby." If they're still uneasy, I offer to see them for an office visit.

FORGETFULNESS—My patients laugh at their forgetfulness late in pregnancy. There is no scientific evidence addressing this point, but I see it all the time. Increasing fatigue and preoccupation with the physical changes of pregnancy or the things to come contribute to this short-term annoyance. Help your partner by writing out sticky notes, fire up the Palm Pilot, or make an extra call to remind her of important appointments (like coming to the obstetrician).

HEARTBURN—A burning sensation in the mid-chest that can radiate upward. It's caused by stomach acid leaking into the lower esophagus. The burning typically gets worse on an empty stomach or when your partner lies down. Don't hesitate to hand her some Tums, encourage her to eat small frequent meals, or prop her head up on pillows while she sleeps. I suggest that women with heartburn take antacids a half hour after each meal and before bedtime. Additional antacids can be taken if symptoms intensify.

Over-the-counter Zantac and Tagamet may be taken for unremitting heartburn. If the discomfort persists, speak with the doctor.

HEMORRHOIDS—Constipation and pressure from the growing uterus cause the rectal blood vessels to protrude from the rectum. Your partner may notice soft lumps around her rectum. They are hemorrhoids. When she moves her bowels, bright red bleeding may occur. Sometimes the blood may be coming from the vagina, not the rectum, so it is important to distinguish where the bleeding is coming from. If she's unsure, placing a mini-pad in her undergarment may help determine the source of the bleeding. Once again, if there are any questions, contact the physician.

Treatment

Over-the-counter hemorrhoid medications

Medicated pads, such as Tucks

Avoid prolonged standing

Soften stools (drink fluid) or take a stool softener, like Colace

Avoid constipation

Occasionally a blood clot can develop in a hemorrhoid, causing severe pain. If home remedies don't work, contact the doctor.

HICCUPS—Your partner may notice sudden, unpredictable movement of the baby. The baby is not having a problem, just the hiccups. Relax! They're a normal pregnancy event.

HOT FLASHES—A sudden, warm flush or heavy sweating can occur throughout the day or night. The flashes can be quite embarrassing and annoying. They are another perfectly normal hassle of the last weeks of pregnancy.

INDUCTION—Triggering the onset of labor with the aid of medication. Induction can be an arduous task, taking up to twenty-four hours, or a relatively quick process, taking just a few hours. Your partner's experience depends on her pelvic exam and how many babies she has had before. Women with prior deliveries or a well-effaced and dilated cervix have a shorter induction.

In some cases, the baby needs to be delivered, but your partner's cervix isn't set for labor (undilated and uneffaced). In order to help reduce the length of labor and risk of cesarean section, medication may be administered to "ripen the cervix." Ripening is the process of helping the cervix efface and dilate prior to the onset of labor. At the present time Cervidil or Misoprostol is the treatment of choice. With either medication, hospitalization is usually suggested to monitor the response to treatment. Cervidil is placed in the vagina and left in place for up to twelve hours prior to induction. It can cause contractions, diarrhea, low-grade fever, or nausea. Misoprostol is taken orally on a fixed schedule for many hours before labor is induced too. If you are lucky, either one will stimulate labor or successfully ripen the cervix.

Some physicians choose other options for "ripening the cervix." They place a urinary catheter or small dilators (laminaria) into the cervix for several hours. Either technique is successful in triggering labor in some patients.

Induction should not be done as a social convenience. It is a medical procedure and should be initiated only when there is a sound medical reason.

Medical reasons to induce:

Overdue pregnancy

High blood pressure

Mom with a medical condition such as heart disease, diabetes, or lupus

Abnormal amount of fluid around the baby

Baby isn't growing well

Poor obstetrical history

Abnormal monitoring tests

We make a big deal about the cervical exam before induction because the rate of cesarean section triples in women with an undilated cervix. Also, we are well aware that an induction can be a long, uncomfortable event. Why subject your partner to a potentially difficult experience (induction) unless there is a good medical reason?

Induction procedure

An intravenous drip of Pitocin is administered to your partner. Over the next several hours the uterus begins to respond with intermittent mild contractions. Eventually the intensity, frequency, and duration of the contractions increase. Once your partner is huffing, puffing, and dilating, she'll be treated like every other woman in labor.

Most couples worry about the pain associated with induction. I tell them that they need a certain number of contractions to deliver the baby. The contractions can happen over six or sixteen hours. With induced labor the contractions tend to be more concentrated but no harder than natural contractions. This makes labor seem more intense. I remind my patients that in a typical labor at home, they would ignore many of the early preparatory contractions by watching television or doing last-minute housework. With induction each contraction shows up on the monitor and is counted by you and your partner. Once labor is established, anesthesia can be offered to alleviate labor discomfort. Speak with your partner's doctor about her/his induction procedure.

INSOMNIA—As your partner's abdomen expands, she'll become more uncomfortable. Trying to find a cozy position to sleep may be nearly impossible. Inopportune baby movements, uterine contractions, and frequent urination contribute to insomnia. The use of a few well-placed pillows may ease the bedtime discomfort.

Acclimating to sleepless nights comes in handy once the baby is born. Who knows? Maybe this is nature's way of preparing your partner for motherhood.

IRRITABILITY—Have you noticed your partner seems more tense or irritable? It goes with the territory. Remember, she isn't sleeping much, she's lugging around a lot of extra weight, and labor is looming. Smile and be patient.

LEG CRAMPS—Leg cramps, especially at night, are very uncomfortable and common. Although we don't know why they happen, I suggest eating bananas (for potassium), taking calcium or magnesium pills, or drinking Gatorade. Getting up and walking around or massaging the sore spot can relieve some of the discomfort too.

LOSS OF URINE—The uterus presses down on the bladder. Standing up suddenly, sneezing, or the baby pushing down can trigger a sudden loss of urine. This becomes a confusing issue when we begin to watch for signs of the amniotic sac breaking.

A safe adage is to evaluate the circumstances surrounding the loss of fluid. Leaking based on straining or standing up suggests that the fluid is urine. If there is a constant leakage of fluid regardless of the position, the amniotic sac may have broken. Call the doctor immediately.

MENSTRUAL CAMPING—Menstrual cramping in the last trimester represents the stretching and widening of the lower part of the uterus in preparation for the big day. The cramps can happen weeks before the onset of labor. If the cramps are severe enough to limit your partner's activity level, check in with the doctor.

NAUSEA—In the last few weeks of pregnancy the uterus begins to press on the stomach, causing nausea. You'll notice your partner's appetite dwindling. For you worriers there is no danger to the baby. Reassure your partner that the baby has grown big enough to reach her stomach. This is a sign of a healthy baby. Encourage her to eat small frequent meals and drink plenty of fluid.

NIGHTMARES—Many women worry about the health of their unborn child. Often this manifests itself in bad dreams. A hug and a pep talk can help ease the maternal instinct to worry.

NONSTRESS TEST (NST)—Any time your partner needs special monitoring to check on the baby's health, it is a "stress" test. In the medical sense, the nonstress test involves monitoring the baby's heart rate to make sure the baby is thriving. The nonstress test is an easy, painless test performed in the doctor's office or hospital.

Indications

Baby growth concern

Decreased fetal movement

Maternal medical conditions

Overdue pregnancy

Physician concern

Poor obstetrical history

Pregnancy-induced diabetes or high blood pressure

Twins, triplets, and beyond

Baby growth concern—A baby growing too slowly or rapidly.

THIRD TRIMESTER

Decreased fetal movement—Anytime the baby fails to meet our movement criteria or seems to be moving less than expected.

Maternal medical conditions—Health problems for the mother such as kidney disease, heart disease, high blood pressure, or systemic lupus erythematosus.

Overdue pregnancy—Pregnancy extending beyond forty weeks.

Physician concern—If the doctor has a bad feeling or is worried.

Poor obstetrical history—Women with a history of a prior stillborn, frequent miscarriage, or having previously delivered a baby much smaller than expected.

Pregnancy-induced diabetes or high blood pressure—Pregnancy complicated by diabetes or high blood pressure

Twins, triplets, and beyond—A multiple pregnancy needs careful fetal monitoring to ensure that all the babies are receiving proper nutrition and oxygen.

Procedure

Your partner is placed on a monitor, and the baby's heartbeat is recorded. During the test, which can take twenty to sixty minutes, the heart rate is monitored and recorded.

Results

> *Reactive*—The heartbeat speeds up by at least fifteen beats for fifteen seconds twice within twenty minutes. This is a healthy baby.

> *Nonreactive*—The heartbeat does not satisfy the criterion for a reactive test.

A nonreactive test can happen when the baby is sleeping, hungry, or the uterus is struggling to provide the baby with enough nutrients.

Before moving on to another type of test, I will give the woman something to eat or a cold glass of water. This may wake up the baby. When all else fails, I use an acoustic stimulator, analogous to an alarm clock, to rouse the baby. After these maneuvers almost all the babies have a reactive test. If the test is still unsatisfactory, I perform an oxytocin challenge test or a special ultrasound (see *Ultrasound* on page 105).

OXYTOCIN CHALLENGE TEST (OCT)—A test of the baby's health that utilizes uterine contractions. It is ordered if the baby does not pass the nonstress test or the physician wants to see how the baby responds to contractions. The OCT is usually performed in a hospital.

Procedure

> An intravenous line is placed in your partner's vein, and Pitocin is administered to stimulate uter-

ine contractions. The contractions are usually quite mild, so your partner doesn't have to worry about "labor pains." The OCT is complete when there are three contractions within ten minutes. It can take between one and four hours to complete. Throughout the test the baby's heart rate is monitored to check its response to contractions. The doctor will evaluate the entire heart-rate strip to make her/his decision on the baby's health.

Results

Negative—The baby's heart rate remained steady or increased in response to three contractions in ten minutes. This is the best result.

Positive—The baby's heart rate dropped after each of the three contractions.

Suspicious—The baby's heart rate drops after some of the contractions, or there were some random drops in the baby's heart rate during the test.

Treatment

Negative—Follow up with the obstetrician for further monitoring, as needed.

Positive—The baby is in a "stress" environment, and delivery should be considered promptly.

Suspicious—Careful follow-up with either a repeat OCT and/or an ultrasound.

If your partner has a placenta previa or prior classical cesarean section, an OCT will not be done.

PAST THE DUE DATE—Only 2 percent of women deliver on their due date. Many first-time mothers go days beyond the due date. With all the discomfort, anxiety, and anticipation associated with the end of pregnancy, waiting becomes a real drag. Everyone is calling, telling your partner she should be delivered. I can't tell you how many patients come in on their due date upset that the baby hasn't arrived. Tell your partner to relax! The end is near. Reassure her that the best way to handle a pregnancy beyond the due date is to let nature do its thing. Along the way the doctor will want to do a nonstress test and pelvic exam. Options will be suggested based on these results and future testing.

Many doctors will wait until forty-one weeks to consider induction with a good pelvic exam and no complications. If your partner is not dilated, careful monitoring will be performed (NST, etc.). By forty-two weeks most babies have delivered. If not, inducing labor is considered. Here are some examples to help you understand.

Examples:

1) 40 weeks pregnant with no problems. Your partner is undilated, uneffaced, and -3 station.

Plan—Count fetal movements, do frequent NSTs, and wait for the onset of labor.

2) 40 weeks pregnant with no problem. Your partner is 2 cm dilated, 100 percent effaced, -1 station.

Plan—Count fetal movements, do frequent NSTs, wait for the onset of labor. Consider induction next week.

3) 40 weeks pregnant with high blood pressure. The exam doesn't matter in this case.

Plan—Consider induction of labor due to high blood pressure.

4) 42 weeks pregnant with no problems. Your partner is undilated, uneffaced, and -3 station.

Plan—Consider induction. *

PELVIC PRESSURE—Has your partner told you she feels the baby is falling out of her vagina? If not, she will soon. Pressure from the baby does intensify as he/she settles down low in the pelvis in preparation for labor. Although the pressure is very uncomfortable, it's not a reliable sign of when labor will begin. My wife was sure the baby was coming three weeks early after feeling an increased pelvic pressure. Four weeks later we had a healthy son.

PRETERM LABOR—Nearly 12 percent of births occur before the thirty-seventh week. They are considered to be preterm. Prematurity is one of the greatest health risks to your baby. Difficulties breathing, feeding, and developing an infection are common in babies born early. By recognizing the signs of preterm labor, we can help prevent the premature birth of many babies.

---

*Some obstetricians will wait beyond forty-two weeks in this case, but they will perform careful fetal monitoring with tests such as the NST, OCT, or a biophysical profile (see *Ultrasound* on page 105) to ensure the baby is getting adequate nutrition and oxygen.

All women experience some mild cramping and contractions later in pregnancy. It may be very difficult to distinguish false labor from the real thing. When I counsel patients on preterm labor, I start off by saying, "If we identify preterm labor early, we have a better chance to stop it." Anytime you have a question about regular contractions before the thirty-seventh week, call.

Risk factors for preterm delivery

History of preterm delivery

Twins, triplets, and beyond

Vaginal bleeding

Cigarette smoking

Prior surgery on the cervix

Vaginal bacteria infection

Unusual-shaped uterus

Illicit drug use

Kidney infection

Signs of preterm labor

Regular, painful uterine contractions—These contractions usually last longer than thirty seconds and come at a regular interval (less than ten minutes apart).

Increasing pelvic pain and pressure— Inordinate pressure, more than before, may be a warning sign of labor. Admittedly, this is a tough symptom to figure out. I have found that many women notice a marked increase in the pelvic pressure in advance of preterm labor.

Increasing vaginal discharge or passage of mucus mixed with blood—Vaginal discharge is common, but a noticeable increase should prompt a call to the doctor. The heavier discharge is the result of contractions pushing secretions out of the uterus.

Leaking watery fluid—Warm fluid gushing or leaking slowly out of the vagina on a constant basis is a sign that the bag of water has broken. When this happens, labor begins within twenty-four hours in most women.

Treatment

Despite all the advances in obstetrics, preterm labor is one of the most difficult problems to treat successfully. The medications don't offer a cure and have very annoying side effects. Our main objective in using them is to slow preterm labor down long enough to give the mom two days of corticosteroid shots if she is under thirty-four weeks pregnant. The shots help protect the premature baby if it delivers early.

In most cases of preterm labor, we don't have advanced warning or the opportunity to give corticosteroids. The patient arrives in active labor and is delivered. In some circumstances we have time to make an initial evaluation to discover the cause of preterm labor. Then we must decide whether to attempt to stop labor or allow the patient to deliver. This can be a tough decision, one requiring the doctor to balance the presumed cause of preterm labor, the risks associated with an early delivery versus the consequences, side effects, and the likely success with treatment.

Delivery of a very premature baby is ideally performed at a hospital with neonatal special-care facilities. Delivery at one of these hospitals gives the premature baby the best opportunity to prosper.

PUBIC BONE PAIN—The pubic bones shift position in preparation for childbirth. They can rub together, creating significant tenderness and discomfort. The pain intensifies while walking around and can be sore to the touch. Warm soaks and decreasing activity are the best ways to ease the pain. After delivery the discomfort dissipates.

RASH—Nearly 2 percent of women will notice a rash. From large raised red spots to small fine dots, they can show up anywhere on the body. Although the spots are typically red, they can also be brown. Itching is the worst symptom and can be very pronounced.

Treatment isn't necessary, but it becomes imperative if the itching is severe. Topical hydrocortisone cream and an Aveeno bath are helpful. If the itch doesn't respond, contact your partner's doctor.

RIB PAIN—Your partner's body recognizes the need to make room for the growing baby to move upward. To do this, her ribs will rotate outward, creating more room. In the process she will experience chest soreness or pain. As long as the pain is mild or intermittent, there's nothing to worry about. Rib pain can also occur when the baby presses or snuggles up under the ribs. This pain goes away when the baby moves. Many of my patients ask if there's a way to coax the baby to change position. Besides lying on the opposite side, the answer is no. The baby does what it wants when it wants. Get used to the idea now because this will be a constant theme over the next eighteen years.

Unrelenting sharp, stabbing rib pain or significant shortness of breath can be a sign of a serious medical condition. Contact the doctor immediately if your partner has either of these symptoms.

RUPTURED MEMBRANES—The amniotic sac holds up to one liter of fluid and can make a nice puddle when it breaks. Nearly 20 percent of women break their water prior to the onset of labor. If your partner notices a gush of warm, clear, odorless fluid or a persistent trickle of fluid running down her leg, it is time to call the doctor. The fluid can be mixed with mucus or blood. If there is a green or brown fluid discharge, call the doctor immediately.

It is important to understand that labor does not always start before or after the membranes rupture. However, three quarters of women will be in labor within twenty-four hours of the bag breaking. Contact the doctor if you have any questions regarding fluid leakage.

SEX—You can be sexually active until your partner's water breaks or labor begins. Don't be surprised if you need to use creative positioning or your partner finds intercourse uncomfortable. Afterward vaginal spotting or uterine cramping may occur. Relax, you haven't hurt your partner or the baby.

Despite the old wives' tales, sex probably does not trigger labor.

SNORING—More than 10 percent of pregnant women snore. Although it may keep you up at night, it is perfectly normal. Encourage her to shift sleeping position to help reduce this nighttime annoyance. If your partner snores and experiences significant daytime sleepiness, she should speak with her doctor.

SORE HIPS—This is another one of the aches and pains associated with your partner's changing shape. Be it after walking or lying down, the hips can ache due to pressure from the baby or the change in her walking pattern. Resting more, walking less, and using a well-placed pillow can ease the discomfort.

SPIDER VEINS—These are swollen, small reddish blood vessels on the legs that are found in clusters or individually. They are unsightly, but don't cause any problems. Most of these veins shrink after pregnancy.

STREP TESTING (GROUP B-STREPTOCOCCUS OR GBS)— Strep is one of a host of bacteria commonly living in the vagina throughout pregnancy. When there is an over-abundance of GBS in the vagina, it can trigger premature birth, premature rupture of the bag of water, or fetal infection. New national guidelines encourage doctors to perform vaginal and rectal cultures on every pregnant woman between the thirty-fifth and thirty-seventh weeks of pregnancy. Those who test positive for this bacteria require antibiotic treatment during labor.

Women who have had strep throat are not at an increased risk of having a baby infected with strep at birth.

STRETCH MARKS—An unavoidable part of growing a baby, stretch marks occur on the breast, thighs, or abdomen. These red, pink, or purple lines are more prevalent later in pregnancy. Although no treatment is successful, many women rub Vitamin E or cocoa butter on their skin.

Unfortunately, stretch marks are permanent, though they blend in with the skin over time. They are one of the lasting memories of childbearing.

SWELLING—Swelling of the feet or hands is very common. In some cases it is hard to imagine that a normal ankle is hidden beneath that puffy exterior. Don't worry! This is not permanent. If your partner props her feet up, reduces her time standing, or wears support stockings, the fluid may ease. However, this annoyance won't go away until after the baby is born. If her hands begin to swell, it is a good time to put her rings in a safe place until after the baby is born. Swelling intensifies during the summertime heat. It's a good idea to invest in air conditioning to help your partner survive the summer.

Many patients are disappointed to discover that their swelling takes several weeks to resolve after delivery. Be patient. The rings will fit again.

TETANUS—If your partner cuts herself on a metal object, she should receive the tetanus vaccine, provided she has not had the shot in the past ten years. It's safe during pregnancy.

TRANSVERSE LIE—An unusual position of the baby where it is lying sideways. These babies can be turned by external cephalic version (see *Breech* on page 78). Babies in the transverse-lie position are always delivered by cesarean section.

TRAVEL—Unforeseen pregnancy complications such as preterm labor become more common later in the pregnancy. Being away from the physician most familiar with your partner's pregnancy can lead to a less-than-optimal result, as well as increased stress and subsequent guilt. Be it for work or pleasure, I discourage travel in the third trimester. A discussion with your partner's doctor can clarify her/his opinion.

If your partner chooses to fly, remind her to move her legs frequently while seated and to always wear her seat belt. The safest and most comfortable place to wear the seat belt is just above her pubic bone.

Most U.S. airlines allow pregnant women to fly up until thirty-six weeks of pregnancy.

TWINS AND BEYOND—More than one baby in the uterus increases the risk of preterm labor and delivery as well as cesarean section. It's important to select a hospital and doctor adept at handling these pregnancies. A few important questions to ask include:

> Does the hospital's nursery handle premature babies?
>
> Does your practice care for twins? Triplets?

Most experienced obstetricians manage twins in their practice. However, due to the many special needs of triplet pregnancies, most obstetricians refer them to specialists in high-risk obstetrics called perinatologists (pair-ee-nay-tall-o-gists).

Compared to a normal pregnancy, twins tend to create more discomfort earlier. Your partner will grow larger, faster, and gain more weight. Every symptom is magnified. Her pregnancy care will be rather uneventful until the end of the second trimester. At that time she will be encouraged to reduce her level of activity and be alert to signs of preterm labor. Over the remaining weeks, frequent ultrasounds will be performed to check the babies' growth. A nonstress test may be ordered as well.

Although many twins are delivered vaginally, there's a tendency toward cesarean section when either baby is in a breech or transverse-lie (lying sideways) position.

ULTRASOUND—The reasons for third-trimester scanning are different from those of earlier scans.

Indications

> Follow-up of earlier ultrasound findings
>
> Check baby's head position
>
> Check the placenta and its location
>
> Evaluate late-pregnancy bleeding
>
> Complement to NST/OCT (biophysical profile)
>
> Discrepancy in fetal growth
>
> Check the amount of fluid surrounding the baby

Follow-up of earlier ultrasound findings— An early ultrasound may have raised questions about the baby that require a follow-up scan. Repeat scanning will help determine if there is a problem. A common example involves a slight swelling in the baby's kidneys. The repeat scan will determine how the kidneys are doing and if they are still swollen.

Check baby's head position—Scanning determines if the baby is head down, breech, or transverse lie (lying sideways.)

Check the placenta and its location—Early scanning may indicate that the placenta is low in the uterus. A repeat ultrasound will check the location of the placenta and exclude a placenta in front of the baby (placenta previa). In addition, ultrasound can assess the health of the placenta by looking for signs of premature aging. This may be a subtle sign of a diminished ability of the placenta to nourish the baby adequately.

Evaluate late-pregnancy bleeding—Ultrasound may detect the cause of bleeding. Sometimes, a placenta previa will be diagnosed. Other times, a placental abruption, premature separation of a portion of the placenta from its attachment to the uterus, can be detected.

Complement to NST/OCT (biophysical profile)—There are instances when the doctor wants to do additional monitoring of the baby. Physicians turn to the biophysical profile for answers. After studying the baby's breathing, movement, tone, and amount of fluid with the ultrasound, a maximum of 2 points are assigned for each studied item. The total is calculated up to 8 points. A score of 6 or higher in conjunction with a reactive NST indicates that the baby is doing well. A lower score may suggest a baby needing further medical attention and possible delivery.

Discrepancy in fetal growth—If the uterus seems to be smaller than expected, ultrasound can be used to evaluate the growth. By measuring the head, thigh bone, and waistline of the baby, we can get a sense of the its size. This helps determine if the baby is living in a healthy, nurturing environment. Repeated scans can be ordered to monitor the growth of the baby over the following weeks. Ultrasound can be used to measure the blood pressure across the umbilical cord too. If the measurement is high, the amount of nutrition and oxygen flowing to the baby is reduced. This may lead to a decline in the baby's growth.

A uterus that is larger than expected can prompt an ultrasound exam to check the amount of water surrounding the baby and its weight. An overabundance of fluid can signal a problem requiring careful monitoring. Other times, the baby is growing larger than expected. The ultrasound can give us an idea of the baby's weight.

Check the amount of fluid surrounding the baby—Scanning can detect insufficient or an overabundance of fluid surrounding the baby. In either instance, close fetal monitoring is required.

VAGINAL BLEEDING—Any bleeding should be carefully monitored. Light bleeding or spotting after intercourse is common. Mucus mixed with blood may be a sign of impending labor (i.e., bloody show). If your partner notices bright red vaginal bleeding or passes blood clots, call the doctor immediately.

VAGINAL BIRTH AFTER CESAREAN SECTION (VBAC)—The adage "Once a cesarean, always a cesarean" has lost its validity over the past decade. Nearly 70 percent of women with a prior cesarean section can have a successful VBAC. Vaginal birth is associated with less post-delivery pain and a faster recuperation than a cesarean section.

For those with a prior cesarean section, it's important to understand the risks associated with a repeat cesarean section (infection, injury to abdominal organs, bleeding, and longer recuperation) and benefits (convenience and prevention of uterine rupture). Recent information has demonstrated that spontaneous labor is associated with a 1 percent risk of uterine rupture, whereas those with certain types of induced labor may increase their risk tenfold. Before making a decision on the type of delivery, I'd evaluate the doctor and hospital to make sure they are able to handle emergencies related to attempting a VBAC.

Ask prospective physicians the following questions:

Is there 24/7 in-hospital anesthesia available?

Does the hospital have 24/7 blood banking available?

Does the doctor encourage VBAC deliveries?

If the answer to any of the questions is no, keep searching! Delivering your baby at the right hospital with the right doctor will make an attempted VBAC very safe!

VAGINAL DISCHARGE—A significant amount of milky white discharge is commonly secreted late in pregnancy.

It is rarely associated with itch or odor. Although it is a nuisance, I would not attempt to treat it.

VAGINAL PAIN—Many women are surprised when they experience sharp, shooting pains in the vagina. The pain can last for several hours and be very intense. It is triggered by the baby pressing on the pelvic nerves. As the baby shifts position, the pain goes away.

VARICOSE VEINS—Your partner may notice the protrusion of veins in her ankle, leg, thigh, or the lips of her vagina. They are varicose veins, caused by a buildup of blood behind the enlarging uterus. The swelling can be painful, but in most instances varicose veins are just unsightly. There are several treatments available.

Treatment

> Avoid prolonged standing
>
> Elevate the leg
>
> Wear support stockings on the affected leg*

Most problems with varicose veins resolve after pregnancy.

In rare cases a blood clot can form in a varicose vein, phlebitis (flee-bye-tis). The leg looks red, swollen, and painful. If your partner is experiencing these symptoms, contact the doctor immediately.

---

*Specially fitted stockings can be ordered by your partner's physician.

THIRD TRIMESTER

WEIGHT—By the third trimester your partner is stunned by how much weight she has gained. She's never weighed this much, and the pounds keep piling on. She might not verbalize her dismay, but she's thinking about it. My best advice is to keep a tight lip. No matter how much weight she has gained, never tease her or, worse yet, mention the word "fat." We don't want her going on a diet. If you're concerned about her weight, speak with her physician. There are some sensible suggestions on ways to limit weight gain.

In the last trimester most women will gain one pound per week. Not all the increase is attributed to food intake. A significant amount of the weight comes from water retention. It shows up as swelling of the feet, hands, or face.

X RAY—Unless absolutely necessary, avoid X ray exposure. When needed, a lead shield can reduce the amount of X ray exposure to the baby. Speak with your partner's doctor if an X-ray is suggested.

PART FOUR

LABOR

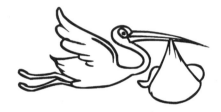

The big day is coming...

LABOR PREPARATION—I can tell you from years of experience that the birth of your baby is the most exciting moment of your life. Despite the grand result, the labor process can be challenging to parents-in-waiting.

From your partner's perspective, she's wondering why she can't see her toes anymore. A quick glance in the mirror is telling her something really big is occupying her belly and it's alive! Her big question is, How is the baby really coming out? She has gone to classes, but the whole process sounds a bit unbelievable, AND everyone she knows, and even strangers, have bombarded her with unsolicited war stories about delivery! All the tales will scare her silly.

You have a totally different take on the things to come. Your partner looks very different; she even acts like someone else. You've gone to class and dared to glance at a heavy-duty maternity book. It all sounds like some B-rated adult movie adventure except you're the costar. Your partner is relying on you to be her strength! Hey, you don't even like to get your blood drawn. This is no time to chicken out. Suck it up and hang tough. She really does need your support and "coaching."

This is a great opportunity to talk about labor, delivery, and what you as a couple want your experience to be. Take a test drive to the hospital. Check how long the drive takes, where you're going in the hospital, and where you should park your car.

Is this labor?

Childbirth classes provide the basic information on the events ahead. The knowledge you've gained will prepare you and is a great source of comfort and empowerment. However, don't try to be your partner's doctor. If you have concerns or questions, don't hesitate to contact the doctor. Remember, she/he can't help unless YOU make the call.

Many patients wonder if classes can really prepare you and your partner? We hope so, but we also know that once nature gets to work, all bets are off. Labor is as unique as the individuals involved. Classes teach you the basics, not how your partner will react to the labor experience. Don't forget the baby has her/his own opinion too. Fortunately, labor is a natural process. With some helpful coaching, you will bring home a beautiful baby and lifelong positive memories.

The following section will help explain some of those vexing terms surrounding labor and delivery.

BLOODY DISCHARGE (SHOW)—Prior to the beginning of labor, some women will expel a bloody, mucous secretion from the vagina. Don't panic. Don't call the doctor just yet. Labor is around the corner but not at hand. Within forty-eight hours many women will be in labor. This discharge should not be confused with the bright red vaginal bleeding that requires an immediate call to the doctor.

FALSE LABOR—Distinguishing real labor from false labor can be a challenge. False labor tends to have short, mild, and more sporadic contractions, as opposed to true labor where the contractions keep getting longer, stronger, and more frequent. I tell my patients that if the contractions are uncomfortable enough to take away their breath or they want to swear, it is a good time to start timing them. When they reach a predetermined frequency (see *Reasons to Call the Doctor Now* on page 114), it is time to contact the doctor.

LABOR

Sometimes I can't tell if a patient is in labor by a phone call. I ask her to take a trip to labor and delivery. While there, your partner will have a pelvic exam and external monitoring of the baby's heart rate and contractions. Only then can labor be truly determined.

It can be tough deciding when to contact the doctor. Having shared three births with my wife, I can sympathize with you. The good news is that we don't expect you to be an obstetrician. When in doubt, call us!

Reasons to Call the Doctor Now

Regular, painful contractions

Vaginal bleeding

Leaking fluid/breaking the bag

Green or brown fluid leaking from the vagina

Constant, severe stomach pain

Maternal exhaustion

Regular, painful contractions—Labor pain is distinctly different from any other type of stomachache or cramp. The uterus becomes tight from top to bottom. A sharp pain, lasting thirty to ninety seconds, is felt in the abdomen or back. The contraction eases up for a period of time before recurring. Monitor the frequency of contractions by recording the interval from the beginning of one contraction to the beginning of the next (not from the end of one contraction to the beginning of the next). Once the contractions occur on a regular basis (depending upon how far you have to drive to the hospital and the doctor's suggestion), it's time to call the doctor.

Vaginal bleeding—Bright red vaginal bleeding merits an immediate call to the doctor. Be ready to go to the hospital at once.

Leaking fluid/breaking the bag—Both a warm gush of fluid leaking from the vagina and/or an intermittent trickle of fluid running down your partner's leg are typical signs of the bag breaking. The fluid should be clear or blood-tinged. Leaking fluid should prompt a phone call to the doctor.

Green or brown fluid leaking from the vagina—Green or brown stained fluid (meconium) leaking from the vagina may indicate the baby is not happy in the uterus. Contact the doctor immediately. Be ready to go to the hospital pronto!

Constant, severe stomach pain—Persistent severe pain may be a sign of the placenta beginning to prematurely separate from the uterus (abruption). Contact the doctor right away and be prepared to go to the hospital now.

Maternal exhaustion—Hours of irregular contractions can lead to sleep deprivation, frustration, and dehydration. Contact the doctor to discuss ways to help your partner.

LABORING AT HOME—Because labor can take many hours, I discourage couples from timing contractions when they are mild and irregular. The early warm-up phase will pass quicker if you and your partner find ways to distract yourselves. Cleaning the house, readying the baby's new room, or watching television are good diversions.

When the contractions become regular and last more than thirty seconds, it's time to start timing them. Based upon your prior discussions with the doctor, a phone call should be made when labor pains are at a predetermined interval, length, and intensity (usually three to five minutes apart, lasting thirty seconds or longer and feeling moderately intense). Don't worry, you will make it to the hospital in plenty of time.

To reduce the discomfort of early labor, women use breathing techniques, walk around the house, blast the shower on the small of their back, or have a back rub. Visualization techniques are also a fine way to deal with labor. Remind your partner to drink clear fluids and refrain from eating hard-to-digest foods once labor begins. Don't forget to eat a little too. I've seen more than a few towering fellows topple over, the victims of hypoglycemia.

Women with complicated pregnancies should speak with their physician regarding the wisdom of laboring at home.

For a woman with a healthy, uncomplicated pregnancy wishing to have a more natural experience, waiting a bit longer at home will shorten her stay in labor and delivery. Make sure to discuss your plans with the doctor in advance so you don't end up being your partner's obstetrician at home!

At the hospital

The following section is based on the common order of events that transpire in the labor and delivery suite.

FETAL MONITORING—

External

Two monitors are placed on your partner's abdomen. One checks the baby's heart rate, while the second records the frequency of uterine contractions. The results are recorded on a strip of paper. By interpreting the information, the frequency of contractions and the baby's general health can be determined.

The baby's heart rate usually fluctuates between 120 to 160 beats per minute. Short episodes above and below this range are common.

The contraction belt registers the frequency of contractions but not their strength.

Internal

In some cases, a monitor may be placed directly on the baby's scalp (fetal scalp electrode) to watch the heart-rate pattern more closely. It's inserted through the vagina during a pelvic exam and doesn't hurt the baby. Using this technology allows a more accurate determination of the baby's health during labor.

If labor slows down, the doctor may insert an internal pressure monitor (intrauterine pressure catheter) to measure the strength of the contractions. This plastic tube is inserted through the vagina and placed in the uterus next to the baby. It does not bother the baby. The monitor tells the doctor the strength of the contractions. If they aren't strong enough, Pitocin can be administered to improve their strength. The internal pressure monitor can also be used like an intravenous line to add fluid to the uterus in case the amniotic fluid is a thick green (meconium) color, the baby's heart rate is dropping, or the doctor feels that there is not enough fluid around the baby.

INTRAVENOUS LINE—In most cases a plastic tube is inserted into your partner's arm to provide fluid to help nourish the baby during labor.

BLOOD TESTS—Blood is drawn, and a complete blood count, blood type, and Rh are done. Other tests may be ordered based upon your partner's medical and obstetrical history.

EVALUATION OF RUPTURED MEMBRANES—If your partner has noticed leakage of fluid, the doctor will perform a speculum examination to obtain a sample of fluid/discharge from the vagina to determine if the amniotic sac has broken. This is done before the pelvic exam.

PELVIC EXAM—A vaginal exam to determine the dilatation, effacement, and station is done.

Effacement—Thickness of the cervix. We describe effacement as a percentage. Zero percent means the cervix is very thick, whereas 100 percent means the cervix is completely thinned out. Effacing is the longest and most tedious part of the labor process. Starting off with a thin cervix bodes well.

Dilatation—The cervix has to stretch open to let the baby pass into the vagina. The measurements go from 0 to 10 centimeters. The process may take many hours, especially when the initial dilatation is less than 5 centimeters. Once the cervix has dilated to 10 cm, delivery is coming soon.

Station—The baby must move down from the pelvis and through the vagina to be delivered. The location of the head in relationship to the middle of the pelvis is referred to as the station. The numbers go from -4 (head floating in the pelvis) to +4 (head coming out of the vagina).

It doesn't matter how much pain or how long your partner has been contracting. Neither of these is an accurate sign of her labor progress. Only a pelvic exam can determine where she stands in the process of labor. Some of my couples are shocked by their progress; some are happy; others are disappointed. For those of you lucky enough to be 5 centimeters and beyond, welcome to the active phase of labor (see *Labor progress* on page 120).

Those less dilated are in the **latent phase** of labor, a time when dilatation may be slow and unpredictable. Your

LABOR

partner may be having booming contractions every two minutes, huffing and puffing, and be 2 centimeters dilated. Two more hours of hard labor, and she may still be 2 centimeters. Before, neither of you believed the books when you read, "Early labor can last up to twenty hours." Now you are living proof.

By understanding the process of labor and the time involved, you'll be able to reassure your partner. Now is the time to earn your title, *Coach*. Take charge. Focus on the positive aspects of labor. Tell her she is doing great and so is the baby. Let her know that you are proud of her. Don't lose sight of the big picture. You are going to be parents very soon.

LABOR PROGRESS—During the active phase of labor, we can make an estimate of the expected delivery time based on known averages for dilatation and pushing.

	Dilatation (cm)/hour	Second Stage (Pushing)
First-time mom	1 cm/hour	2 hours
Second-time mom and beyond	1.5 cm/hour	1 hour

Once your partner reaches 10 centimeters, it is time for the second stage of labor. PUSHING is hard work, can take several hours, and requires a great coach!

Examples of predicted time to normal delivery

First baby

> Patient is dilated 5 cm
>
> 5 hours x 1 cm/hour = 5 cm (to 10 cm)
>
> + 2 hours pushing
> _____
>
> 7 hours until delivery

Second baby

> Patient is dilated 5 cm
>
> 3 to 4 hours x 1.5 cm/hour = 4.5 to 5 cm (to 10 cm)
>
> + 1 hour pushing
> _____
>
> 4 to 5 hours until delivery

SLOW PROGRESS—If the contractions are spacing out or less intense, the rate of dilatation will slow down. In this situation the doctor may add Pitocin to strengthen and increase the frequency of contractions. She/he might also insert a pressure catheter into the uterus to monitor the strength and frequency of the contractions. The ultimate goal of Pitocin is to help labor progress safely.

PAIN MANAGEMENT—Labor is synonymous with discomfort. Finding effective means to contend with the hours of labor contractions is one of the focal points of prepared childbirth and Lamaze classes. After helping thousands of couples navigate through labor, I can offer you one major piece of advice. Be open-minded about pain management during labor. There is no way to anticipate how your partner will react to the contractions or how long labor will take. She may be exhausted from being up all night or very sensitive to labor pain. It's all right to manage the pain. And you should be your partner's number one supporter in this regard. I cannot emphasize this point enough. Your partner wants your approval and support! Give it to her. Forget about your preconceived notions. Nobody really cares if your partner did it naturally or not. Everyone just wants to see a healthy, happy baby and mom.

Don't worry about making the choices alone. The doctor and nurse will be there to help you make the best decisions.

BREATHING—A systematic technique to cope with labor pain was perfected by a French obstetrician named Fernand Lamaze. Through breathing, he was able to help women avoid the sedation and narcotic usage commonly administered through the 1960s to deal with labor pain. Instead, women were able to take charge of their pain and have a "natural birth." His techniques continue to be used effectively and are the basis of present-day Lamaze childbirth classes.

WALKING—Walking can ease the discomfort associated with labor. Some doctors feel it helps speed early labor. Don't expect your partner to be trotting around when she's in active labor. Most of the time, she'll prefer to lie down.

BACK MASSAGE—Rubbing the lower back vigorously can ease labor pain, especially "back labor." Some of my patients have their partner roll a tennis ball over their lower back during contractions.

TENS **(TRANSCUTANEOUS ELECTRICAL NERVE STIMULATOR)**—A device creating an electrical current that is attached to pads placed on specific spots on the back. By increasing the current, labor pain can be reduced. Special arrangements are needed to procure one of these devices. After checking with your partner's physician, contact a local physical therapist to learn how to use the unit and obtain one for labor and delivery.

NARCOTICS—Long the standard for managing labor, narcotics have fallen out of favor because of their sedating effects on mother and baby. However, they still have a role in selected cases. Demerol, Morphine, Stadol, and Nubain are a few of the medications used in labor and delivery units across the United States.

EPIDURAL—The most significant change in childbirth in the last thirty years has been the advent of the epidural. Safe and effective, the epidural is the ultimate pain management tool. The procedure involves placing a small plastic tube in the low back. Once inserted, local anesthetic medication is injected, numbing the nerves that sense the pain of labor. Your partner's discomfort will dissipate quickly. Instead of labor pain, she'll be very comfortable, experiencing numbness and slight uterine tightness or mild pelvic pressure. After hours of discomfort, easing the pain is a great relief. Many women become so relaxed that they take a well-deserved nap. Most hospitals utilize a continuous drip of the local anesthetic through the epidural, providing relief until the baby's delivery is complete.

Some hospitals do not offer epidural anesthesia. Others provide epidural anesthesia during limited hours, when an anesthesiologist is available, or when your partner is dilated a certain number of centimeters. In these situations your partner may have to go through many hours of labor before becoming a candidate for an epidural. Speak with your partner's physician regarding her/his rules for the use of epidural and the hospital's policy as well.

If an epidural is an important option for your partner, ask the doctor a few simple questions up front.

> Does the hospital offer 24/7 epidural anesthesia?
>
> When do you allow your patients to have an epidural?*
>
> Is there a specific doctor assigned to provide epidural anesthesia exclusively during the day and night?**

If you don't like the answers, look for a hospital that provides the services you want.

---

*Many physicians have a minimum dilatation before they will allow your partner to receive an epidural.

**In many hospitals the anesthesiologist assigned to administer epidural anesthesia is working in the operating rooms as well as covering the labor unit. Your partner may have to wait several hours to receive an epidural.

Frequently I'm asked if inserting an epidural hurts. I reply, "Not half as much as one contraction." This is the absolute truth. Having an epidural is safe and effective. It has taken the pain and fear out of childbirth. Instead of focusing on hours of labor pains, laboring women and their partners can look forward to the birth of their new addition.

Those who oppose the use of an epidural will warn you about the side effects, which include headache, infection, prolonged numbness of a specific nerve, backache, or failure to alleviate the pain entirely. They will probably tell you that it slows down labor too. This is a misleading statement. While it is true that labor contractions may slow down once and epidural is given, a small dose of Pitocin will get labor right back on track, pain-free.

They will also tell you that an epidural reduces your partner's sense of pressure when it's time to push. This is true. Your partner won't have intense rectal pressure, and it might take a bit longer to deliver the baby. To obstetricians, this is just fine. I have found that with good nursing and coaching, the baby will make its arrival on time.

PUSHING—Once the cervix has dilated to 10 centimeters, it's time to push the baby out. With or without an epidural, your partner will feel like she has to move her bowels. Admittedly, those without an epidural will feel much more pressure, but both will know something is different.

Pushing requires a coordinated effort, synchronizing the peak of contractions with a strong pushing effort on behalf of the laboring woman. The exact length of this stage of labor varies from minutes to hours. A nurse will work with you and your partner to help push the baby out.

Most first-time moms push for one to two hours. Subsequent pregnancies are rewarded by a much shorter pushing phase.

FORCEPS/VACUUM—The physician may choose to conclude the pushing phase because the baby isn't tolerating labor, your partner has been pushing for a prolonged period of time, or she's unable to continue pushing. In these situations it's reasonable to assist with the birth. The doctor will chose either forceps or vacuum. While each method is very safe, the decision will be based on the individual physician's expertise with the equipment.

> *Forceps*—Although these metal tongs look like salad spoons, they have been carefully crafted to fit the mother's pelvis and baby's cheeks safely. Once in position, gentle traction is applied to the forceps while the mom is pushing. The forceps are released once the baby's head is delivered. The baby may have crease marks around its cheeks from the spot where the forceps were resting. The marks disappear within a few days.

> *Vacuum*—A plastic cup utilizing suction to help deliver the baby. The device is placed over the baby's scalp, and in conjunction with the mother's

pushing, gentle traction is applied. The baby's head will have a more pronounced cone shape than normal. With a hat on your baby's head and a few days extra, the baby will look just like you!

DELIVERY—Pushing will bring the baby down the birth canal and, with the guidance of the pelvic muscles, angle the baby for its exit. The baby's head will begin to separate the lips of the vagina and be visible between contractions (crowning). Your partner may experience significant pelvic pressure during this short interval. She may describe it as having to move her bowels. With each ensuing contraction, the head stretches the opening. When the baby is just about ready to be born, the doctor may opt to cut an episiotomy (see *Episiotomy* on page 128) to prevent tearing and give the baby more room to exit.

Amazing things will begin to happen as you watch the baby's head pop out, followed by the shoulders twisting and turning to make their entrance. The chest, umbilical cord, genitals, and legs follow quickly.

Congratulations! Get the camera fired up and shoot a few tasteful photos.

Once the baby has arrived, his/her nose and mouth will be suctioned as the doctor and nurse make a quick assessment of the baby's overall health. After the umbilical cord is clamped and cut, the baby will be wrapped in a blanket to stay warm. **Apgar scores** will be assigned at the first and fifth minute of life. This score indicates the baby's

LABOR

general health and is based on the baby's breathing, muscle tone, reflexes, color, and heart rate. Most babies receive a score of 7 or above.

While you're marveling at your new addition, cord blood can be obtained and saved for your newborn or for donation (see *Cord blood collection* on page 81). Next the placenta is delivered. Compared to the baby, it almost falls out. The doctor will check your partner carefully, making sure everything has been delivered and determining the need to sew up an episiotomy. Additional scraps and tears will be identified and repaired at the same time. Most new moms will need a few stitches.

EPISIOTOMY—A surgical incision cut from the opening of the vagina and toward the rectum. It helps protect the vagina from excessive trauma, muscle damage, and eases the baby's delivery. The decision to make an episiotomy is based on the ability of the vaginal opening to stretch and the size of the baby. The incision isn't made until the baby's head has stretched the vaginal tissue to its limit. Shortly thereafter the baby is born. The episiotomy is stitched up with the benefit of an anesthetic (local or epidural). Within several weeks of birth the stitches melt away.

Does everyone need an episiotomy? Of course not! However, most first-time moms have an episiotomy because the tissue has never been stretched before.

CESAREAN SECTION—The surgical delivery of the baby through an abdominal incision.* Cesarean sections may be scheduled in advance or may be an emergency. The decision to deliver by cesarean section is based upon the position of the baby (breech or transverse lie), the progress of your partner's dilatation, and how well the baby is tolerating labor, as indicated by the fetal heart monitor.

After an epidural, a spinal, or general anesthesia is administered, the cesarean section is performed. At many hospitals the father-to-be is encouraged to be present for the surgery unless his partner is having general anesthesia. If you are squeamish, as most dads are, you don't have to watch the surgery. You can sit next to your partner, safely hidden behind a surgical drape. Most physicians will let you know when the baby is about to be born. I'd strongly recommend standing up and welcoming your new addition. You'll be glad you did!

While your baby is being cleaned up, the doctor will complete the surgery.** In recovery, your partner will greet her baby.

---

*Nearly 25 percent of all births are by cesarean section.
**Most cesarean sections are completed within sixty minutes.

Closing

In closing, I offer you and your partner Pickles and Ice Cream: A Father's Guide to Pregnancy as a handy guide to the ABC's of pregnancy. Refer to it often and feel free to follow up with your partner's doctor with any further questions. I wish you much success as a father-in-waiting and someday father. It is the most important—and the best—job you will ever have.

Here are a few parting thoughts to stay in your partner's good graces throughout this tumultuous time.

Your partner is never fat. She is pregnant.

Reassure her when she has doubts.

Be tolerant when she is crabby or tired.

Give her a back massage with and without her prompting.

Give her a hug often.

Remind her of the great job she is doing.

Show a genuine interest in the pregnancy.

Meet the doctor.

Go to childbirth classes.

Be the best coach you can be.

Share this nine-month adventure with your partner.

ABOUT THE AUTHOR

Craig Bissinger is a highly respected, board-certified obstetrician and gynecologist. During his twenty-year career, Dr. Bissinger has delivered over 5000 babies and guided thousands of couples through the nine-month adventure of pregnancy. He has a busy obstetrics and gynecology practice in northwest New Jersey.

Dr. Bissinger completed his residency in obstetrics and gynecology at Rush-Presbyterian St. Luke's Medical Center in Chicago, Illinois, where he was selected as the administrative chief resident. He has continued his interest in education, giving lectures on a variety of health topics in the community and to professional groups. He is a teacher and lecturer, having taught medical students and residents from Columbia University College of Physicians and Surgeons, Harlem Hospital, Roosevelt Hospital, and the University of Medicine and Dentistry, New Jersey, on an ongoing basis as part of his lifelong commitment to training the next generation of doctors.

Dr. Bissinger is a medical expert and frequent contributor to the Fisher-Price website, as well as the past editor and author of numerous articles for Healthology.com's pregnancy section. He has been a contributor to ABC.com. While waiting for babies to be delivered, Dr. Bissinger has written two, as of yet, unpublished medical thrillers: *Ill-Conceived* and *Deadly Medicine*.

Dr. Bissinger is married to his lovely wife, Margie, and is the proud father of Josh, Scott, and Lindsey.

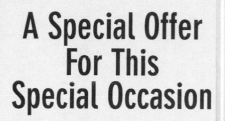